SIMON & SCHUSTER

NEW YORK   LONDON   TORONTO   SYDNEY   SINGAPORE

Brea

A Guy's Guide to Pre

the

ancy · **Mason Brown**

ILLUSTRATIONS BY JOE OESTERLE

SIMON & SCHUSTER
Rockefeller Center
1230 Avenue of the Americas
New York, NY 10020

Designed by Karolina Harris
Manufactured in the United States of America

10 9 8 7 6 5 4 3 2 1

Library of Congress Cataloging-in-Publication Data
ISBN 0-7432-1970-8
Brown, Mason.
Breathe : a guy's guide to pregnancy / Mason Brown.
p. cm.
1. Pregnancy—Popular works. 2. Pregnancy—Humor. 3.Pregnant women—Relations
with men. I. Title.

RG526 .B76 2002
618.2'4—dc21   2001049983

For information regarding special discounts for bulk purchases, please contact Simon & Schuster
Special Sales at 1-800-456-6798 or business@simonandschuster.com

It is a sad comment on our society that a book as artfully crafted and well meant as this requires a dis-
claimer. Nevertheless, if you haven't already suspected, then you're about to find out for sure that "this
publication is sold with the understanding that the author and publisher are not engaged in rendering
medical, health, or any other kind of personal or professional services in the book." Far from it, "you
should consult a competent professional before adopting any of the suggestions in this book."

If you are so foolish as to disregard the above mentioned notice, "the author and publisher specifically
disclaim all responsibility for any liability, loss, or risk, personal or otherwise, which is incurred as a
consequence, directly or indirectly, of the use and application of any of the contents of this book,"
though if you do, you probably deserve what you've got coming to you.

Acknowledgments

This book could not have come about if it hadn't been for one very special person. Me. I'd like to thank myself for always being there, except for that one time in Vegas. What the hell was I thinking?

I'd also like to thank Geoff Kloske at Simon & Schuster for encouraging me to start a family as research for a "spec" humor book. And, of course, thanks to Karen, John, and Alison, who have suffered so much as a result of Geoff's terrible vision.

Others who made invaluable contributions include: Joe Oesterle, Nicole Graev, Paul Blevins, Professor Larry Fignon, Nancy and Susan Kesmodel, the Krumenaker twins, Tom Rhodes, George Ruiz, Jasmine St. Claire, Dr. T. Berry Brazelton, and those chicks from the "What to Expect" books.

Most of all, I'd like to thank my father, who used none of the techniques described in this book.

To John and Alison.

At least you won't have to go into psychotherapy unarmed.

Contents

A Word from the Doctor

People who hear my name for the first time often think I'm a doctor. I'm not. I have no medical training whatsoever. But my friends call me "The Doctor" because of the way I smooth talk the ladies. I can really operate. As for bona fide medical expertise, let me make myself perfectly clear—I can barely tell my head from my asshole.

In fact, I had nothing to do with writing this book. Mason Brown wrote the book, and he called me up because he needed someone to write a foreword. When it comes to parenting, if I'm a father, I sure as hell don't know about it. And I don't want to know either.

From the desk of Jimmy "The Doctor" Savante
March 2001

A Word from the Author

The creation of a book is much like giving birth. Just like a mother, an author must nurture and feed an entity growing inside him—alien yet wholly his own. Just like a mother, cravings develop, though rather than pickles and ice cream, most authors desire cigarettes and cheap gin. And just like a mother, an author will not lift heavy objects during the gestation period. Unlike his maternal counterpart, however, an author will refrain from heavy lifting long after publication, whereas a mother will be expected to at least pick up her child.

Yet at the end of it all, authors and mothers are both rewarded for their pains. Mothers with their babies, and authors—well, let's just say that I wish each and every one of you could experience the giddiness I feel when providing the world with a shoddily-bound paperback that's one step away from pornography.

Mason Brown
Santa Monica, California

Introduction

The world is filled with books that help women deal with the changes they undergo during pregnancy. Often these books deign to include a sidebar or two about the man, but for the most part he is immediately relegated to the status of his wife's personal assistant. To be sure, any man in a relationship should be used to "drone" status, but somehow pregnancy makes it seem more definitive.

Worse than that, the father-to-be has no guidebook that tells him what to expect. His wife's books tell her she should be eating folic acid, but what should he be eating? She knows that she should take a light walk every day, but should he walk, too? Or is walking a pansy-ass exercise no matter how you slice it? A young father may feel helpless, or even guilty (especially if he still finds himself looking at pictures of lovely, young Swedish au pairs).

This book is designed with you, the father, specifically in mind. It follows the course of the pregnancy and gives you step-by-step advice about what will be happening to YOU be-

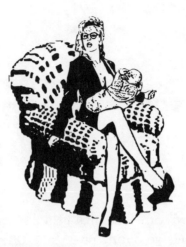

fore, during, and after your wife's pregnancy. And stop looking
at that au pair! What's wrong with you! You're going to be a father, for crying out loud!

You make me sick.

1

Getting Started

Getting started seems simple. Have some eggs, some tuna, plenty of rest, and watch Traci, I Love You *with your wife. Then bang away like a summer stock production of* Stomp.

But hold on there, sport. Are you sure you're ready to be a dad? Are you sure she's ready to be a mom? What if you're having trouble getting her pregnant? How can you tell if you've succeeded?

Don't think that just because you've surfed the Internet for porn, you know the score about fatherhood. After all, were you searching for pictures of pregnant *naked women? Please tell me the answer is no.*

One

On Deciding to Become a Father

Unlike marriage, fatherhood is not something to be entered into lightly or unadvisedly. You must understand the full range of responsibilities and duties it entails. Having a baby is a full-time job. You've got to feed it, clothe it, shelter it. I mean, man, that's a lot of hassle.

So before you embark on fatherhood, make a list of reasons why you want to have a child. Compare your reasons with the following list:

GOOD REASONS TO BECOME A DAD

- You and your wife have discussed having a family, and the time just seems "right."
- You love the idea of fatherhood, with all the joys and responsibilities it entails.
- You want to teach, love, and nurture a precious, tiny human.

BAD REASONS TO BECOME A DAD

- You hated your dad, and you want to take it out on someone.
- Just to see if your boys can swim.
- To win a bet.
- You think it will make you look more mature.
- Everybody else is doing it.

Still think you're ready? Many high schools require their sex-ed students to care for a plastic doll for two weeks in order to help illustrate the full-time nature of parenting. Why don't you try it? If your "test" baby looks like this, then maybe you should hold off on having children—at least for a little while.

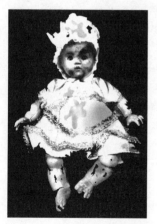

If, however, you passed the baby doll test (or, more likely, figured, "Who the hell has time to drag around a stupid plastic doll?" and decided not to bother), you might still want to test your "Fatherhood Aptitude" by taking the following test.

Use a number 2 pencil. 30 minutes

The Fatherhood Aptitude Test
Multiple Choice

1. The best way to calm a crying baby is to:
   a. hand him off to mommy.
   b. gently rock him up and down.
   c. slap him silly.

2. An appropriate baby-sitter is:
   a. one of our relatives.
   b. a trusted teenage daughter of a friendly neighbor.
   c. an English au pair.
3. Which of the following is an acceptable toy for a baby?
   a. A large doll with plastic crinkle-paper stuffing.
   b. A large, hard, plastic teething ring.
   c. A large, plastic dry-cleaning bag.
4. Which of the following best describes your reasons for wanting to become a father?
   a. I love kids.
   b. I feel the time is right to have a family.
   c. I enjoy playing with my Tamogotchi hatch-an-egg video game.
5. Why do you think you'd make a good father?
   a. I'm so hopelessly, deliriously in love with my wife, that my happiness can't help but rub off on our child.
   b. I look forward to imparting all of my skills to a future generation.
   c. I just finished reading Earl Woods' book *Training a Tiger.* I'm ready to get started immediately.
6. Your wife wants to start trying to have a baby. She's charted her temperature, and knows that she's been ovulating on a twenty-nine-day cycle. If today is March 10, and her temperature last peaked five days ago, when is the best time to try to conceive?
   a. April 4.
   b. April 5.
   c. Right now. Continue trying until my Viagra runs out.

7. Baby : Beer ::

   a. Square Pegs : Round Holes

   b. Checks : Stripes

   c. Who the hell let the baby near my beer? That's *my* beer, dammit!

8. You hope that your first child is:

   a. a Girl.

   b. a Boy.

   c. other.

9. The young father picked up his newborn baby with _____ in his eyes and gently _____.

   a. love . . . sang a lullaby.

   b. joy . . . Cooed nonsense syllables.

   c. horror . . . dropped it.

10. By the end of its second month, a baby should be able to:

   a. smile.

   b. respond to a bell in some way, such as startling, crying, or quieting.

   c. read.

11. goo goo : ga ga ::

   a. boo boo : ba ba

   b. Milli : Vanilli

   c. Shut : Up

12. Four babies are getting weighed in the maternity ward. Your baby, R, weighs more than V. T weighs less than R. S weighs more than V but less than T. Which of the following is the correct lineup of babies from smallest to biggest?

   a. V, S, T, R.

   b. Cannot be determined from the information given.

   c. Which one is mine, again?

True or False?

1. Babies can eat Doritos.

   T   F

2. Babies can be left unattended if you are pretty darn sure you will return by the end of the hour.

   T   F

3. Babies can't scream very loudly since they just have tiny, little baby lungs.

   T   F

4. Once you have a baby, you will have more free time since there will be extra hands around the house.

   T   F

5. Baby fat insulates babies from all but the coldest arctic conditions.

   T   F

6. You will still be able to golf on weekends after the baby is born.

   T   F

7. Most pregnant women look like Hunter Tylo.

   T   F

8. I plan on videotaping the birth and then showing it to friends.

   T   F

9. I was born a rambling man.

   T   F

10. Someday, I would like to appear on the *Jerry Springer Show*.

    T   F

11. Lamaze breathing techniques could also be useful when I'm on the can.

    T   F

12. Whenever you mention that you'd like to have a large family of, say, five kids, your wife anxiously eyes the bathtub.

    T   F

Short Essay:

What does commitment mean to you?

Stop!!

If you have finished before the time allotted, you may go over any questions in this section. Then place your answer sheet facedown in front of you with your pencil on top. Do not go on to any additional sections. Do not run screaming out the door to a seedy singles bar for casual, anonymous sexual encounters.

Scoring

If you answered any of the questions, you pass. And if by some miracle of nature you actually tried to write an essay, then you've got definite fatherhood potential (unless you wrote "all work and no play makes Jack a dull boy" over and over again, in which case don't go on any vacations in the north woods with your family).

Note: If you answered "c" to any of the multiple choice questions, or "True" to any of the True/False questions, then beware! You are a moron. Of course, that alone does not disqualify you from fatherhood in any way.

Trying to Get Pregnant

G etting pregnant doesn't just happen. You have to work at it (unless you're dating an unwed teen, in which case pregnancy can occur via contact with a doorknob).

Amazingly enough, science has proved beyond doubt that the odds of conception are inversely proportional to the desirability of conception. A simple graph renders this concept easy to grasp.

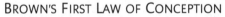

BROWN'S FIRST LAW OF CONCEPTION

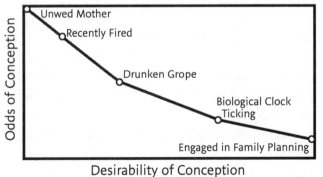

This immutable law of nature results in a curious corol-lary—the more financially successful a couple is, the more likely they are "trying" to have a baby. "Trying to have a baby" is a euphemism for "rogering like feral weasels," which is in turn a euphemism for "having sex often."

Some couples proudly announce that they are trying to have a baby without realizing that they are presenting an unsavory visual picture to their audience, who immediately conjure up the image of the naked wife doing a headstand while her husband cheers his mighty swimmers onward. More often than not, this visual image is uncannily accu-rate.

Still others try to conceal their efforts, feeling that failure to conceive reflects badly on themselves. Unfortunately for these shy souls, it is all too easy to tell when a couple is really mak-ing an effort. In such cases, one or more of the following symptoms will appear:

FOR THE MAN
- Drowsiness
- Irritability
- Heightened desire to watch *SportsCenter*

FOR THE WOMAN
- Normal post-coital glow replaced by grim attitude of sol-dier in the trenches
- Constant concern over husband's choice of briefs rather than boxers
- Neck strain from standing on her head after sex

Obviously, if a couple would really, truly make good parents, then all efforts to conceive are rendered futile. Nature abhors functional families. So, if you really want your wife to get pregnant, forget fertility clinics—institute divorce proceedings. Just remember to have one last drunken, abusive fling before separating. You'll be a daddy in no time.

Improving Your Chances of Conception

Of course, you may wish to have kids and yet not want to turn into an abusive drunk. That's okay. Just remember, it may take a little more effort to succeed. But don't give up hope. There are a variety of methods guaranteed to improve your chances of becoming a father.

LOWERING TESTICULAR TEMPERATURE

A high testicular temperature lowers a man's sperm count. Women who wish to get pregnant often become obsessed with this peculiar fact. It is the one pregnancy variable that they can control, so they'll be damned if your testicles aren't frosty cold. While amusing at first, their concern soon becomes annoying at best and downright unpleasant at worst. More than one prospective father has woken up on a hot summer evening only to find his wife trying to surreptitiously slip his testicles into a jug of ice water.

Many couples go through a boxers vs. briefs argument, eventually surmising that boxers let more air circulate about the testes. Some women go so far as to insist on mesh boxers, available only in gay specialty stores. The ideal male undergarment, from the prospective mother's point of view, would be a finely calibrated thermo-regulatory device fashioned out of readily available household items.

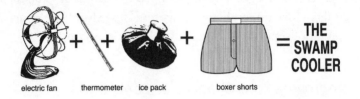

electric fan   thermometer   ice pack   boxer shorts

The best response is to make your wife's obsession work for you. Properly handled, your testicles can provide you with a variety of pleasing benefits:

- You no longer have to do yard work. It's hot out there. Imagine the furnace that would be your nutsack if you should have to mow the lawn.
- What better way to keep cool than with a constant supply of frosty beverages? But God forbid your testicles get overheated while running for refreshment. Let the wife do it.
- Exercise??? Are you mad??? Why not just shoot my unborn child right now???

In Vitro Fertilization

Not all sperm are strong swimmers. But just because you're shooting little minnows instead of mighty salmon, don't think that your boys can't make it upstream. Heck no! Doctors can take a sample of your sperm, extract an egg from your wife, and ensure that they get together by swishing them around in a test tube. Then, they can implant the fertilized egg in the womb.

The extraction and implantation of the egg is a painful and complicated procedure. But guess what? It doesn't concern you. That's her problem. What you *do* have to worry about is the collection of your sperm sample.

The typical collection process consists of a nurse leading you to a room (the "masturbatorium") and handing you a cup. You are meant to emerge several minutes later and depart unobtrusively. But it doesn't have to be so clinical. I mean, when else are you going to be encouraged to masturbate in a doctor's office in the middle of the day. Take your time. Enjoy yourself.

In fact, most fertility doctors keep a small stock of adult magazines and videos for men who are having trouble. Make sure you are one of these men. Insist that you see their entire library. Ask for deviant marital aids (leather chaps, vacuum pumps, vibrating nipple clamps, etc.—heck, make them work). Milk it for all it's worth. Who knows, if you're really struggling, they might even send in the head nurse. The most amazing part? Your wife will congratulate you when you're done!

WONDER DRUGS

Fertility "wonder" drugs stimulate the release of extra eggs during a woman's cycle, thereby increasing the chances that sperm will reach at least one of the eggs. If multiple eggs are fertilized, this in turn increases the odds of successful implantation onto the uterine wall. Of course, if everything works out perfectly, multiple fertilized eggs may successfully implant themselves.

Indeed, thanks to the miracle of modern medicine, septuplets are now a reality. Why not go for the record? Administer as many fertility pills as possible. If you hit octuplets, diaper companies will probably throw in free Huggies for the first year. Of course, if you only have quadruplets, then you are on the hook for a fortune.

SURROGATE MOTHERS

Surrogate mothers are an option if (a) your wife has medical reasons preventing her from giving birth, or (b) your wife decides to simply rent a womb instead of going through the painful process herself.

Even in our current free market economy, however, option (a) is usually the only one permitted by law. Also, women who want a surrogate mother just for the sake of convenience also tend to want nannies to rear their child for them, because looking after a kid is hard work. In other words, these women are thinking just like men. Pretty much would make you a gay fellow if you were married to an option (b) woman, wouldn't it?

But assuming your wife needs a surrogate mother for reasons unrelated to her career goals, then by all means think about it. Just don't get too excited. You don't get to have sex with the surrogate mother. It's the same old "go into a cup" routine as in vitro fertilization.

Let's dispel a few common myths about surrogacy:

- It's not cheap. Typically a surrogate mother costs at least twenty thousand dollars or more.

- Surrogate mothers do not invariably end up suing for custody of the children. (Key word: "invariably.")
- Surrogate mothers are not all kinky Swedish babes who want to insinuate themselves into your marriage.
- The woman you are having an affair with is NOT a surrogate mother.
- Crack whores do NOT make good surrogate mothers.
- If a strange man offers to fellate you at the Walt Whitman rest stop off the New Jersey Turnpike and you accept, that's not surrogacy. It's anonymous gay sex.
- Despite the scientific-sounding name, if your wife hires a "surrogate father," that still makes you a cuckold.

BREEDING AN ARMY OF CLONES

Combine wonder drugs, in vitro fertilization, and surrogate mothers and what do you get? Well, if the idea of breeding an army of clones doesn't leap out at you, then you'll never rule the world thanks to twisted genetic experiments gone horribly awry. The math is really very simple. Figure twenty thousand dollars per surrogate mother, each of whom bears seven bioengineered clones. For a mere 1 million dollars, you are well on your way to a full battalion of 350 identical super soldiers! The old saying certainly is true: "There has never been a better time in the world to be a demented scientist filled with insane hubris."

ADOPTION

The only surefire way to have a kid is to adopt. But even that can take too long. If you want a kid right away, then you'll need to go through the black market. While you might be appalled at the idea of buying a child at first, you'll soon find that so-called white slaver's prices can be quite reasonable.

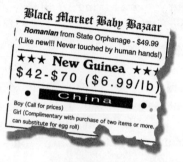

Black Market Baby Bazaar

Romanian from State Orphanage - $49.99
(Like new!!! Never touched by human hands!)

★★★ **New Guinea** ★★★
$42-$70 ($6.99/lb)

China

Boy (Call for prices)
Girl (Complimentary with purchase of two items or more.
can substitute for egg roll)

If you can't afford the money but still want to get a top quality baby, don't despair. With the proper planning and a little bit of luck, there are still plenty of ways to become an adoptive parent. Just keep your eyes open. Good sources of babies include:

- Ladies' rooms at high school proms
- Cars getting rolled into lakes
- Internet chat rooms
- Milk cartons (finders, keepers!)
- The reeds along the banks of the River Nile

KEEPING A GOOD THING GOING

Of course, some men find that trying to have a baby turns out to be the most sex they have in their life, and they want to keep riding that train for as long as they can. Their problem is just the opposite. How do they keep having sex without actually impregnating their spouse?

Obviously, the best way to keep trying without succeeding is to disable your sperm delivery system. Have a vasectomy. She'll never know. The problem is you may want kids sometime in the future and, well, too bad. Also, if your wife finds out that you've snipped your sperm chutes, then you're in for a world of pain. A much easier method: Right before penetration, say, "look over there!" and surreptitiously slip on a condom.

Other solutions involve controlling sperm production. Just as lowering the temperature of your testicles creates hardy, active sperm, raising the temperature creates lazy tropical conditions leading to "siesta sperm." There are several recommended ways to achieve the desired temperature:

- Wear a fur-lined jockstrap (a "nut-muffler").
- Insist on foreplay in the jacuzzi.
- Buy scalding hot coffee at a McDonald's drive-thru. Hold cup tightly between thighs. Spill.

The final proven method of birth control is to masturbate like a sex-crazed colobus monkey. Do it every hour, on the hour. By the end of each day, you'll be lucky if you're dry firing. On the downside, a day or two of sessions like this and you'll almost certainly start to find your desire to have constant sex waning. In fact, getting her pregnant will sound like welcome relief from the hell you've been going through.

The "masturbation method" (as it's called by the Roman Catholic Church) works for all men over twenty. If you're a teenager, it has no useful effect whatsoever, as nature has compensated for this purely normal activity by constantly producing approximately thirty billion sperm an hour for the average, horny seventeen-year-old male. Approximately.

Three

Are You Pregnant?

N o.

You're a man. Men can't get pregnant, you moron!

Some men, however, experience what is known as "empathic pregnancy." They feel symptoms that mimic actual pregnancy signals. Other men get bad gas. The point is, even if you feel like you are pregnant, don't worry about it. You're not.

Here is a table of common "empathic pregnancy symptoms," along with their actual cause:

COMMON EMPATHIC PREGNANCY SYMPTOMS

SYMPTOM	POSSIBLE CAUSE	WHAT IT IS NOT
Weight Gain	Overeating. You could be getting fat.	Pregnancy.
Morning Nausea	Binge drinking. Sometimes known as a "hangover."	Pregnancy.
Your Skin Glows	Sweating. Eating greasy foods.	Pregnancy.
Missed Period	Don't worry about it, champ.	How many times do I have to say—YOU'RE NOT PREGNANT?
Paired with Danny De Vito in horrible "science gone awry" comedy about juiced-up Austrian weight-lifter getting pregnant	Bad Agent.	It's only makeup. You're not pregnant.
Giving birth to a child.	You're a woman, you moron!	It can't be anything else. That's how things work!

Is She Pregnant?

Well, usually she'll tell you. Then she'll get fat. Then she'll give birth. If these three things occur, you will know with certainty that she was pregnant.

Sometimes, however, women show signs of pregnancy that are actually symptoms of something else.

POSSIBLE SIGNS THAT YOUR WIFE IS PREGNANT

SIGN	WHEN IT APPEARS	OTHER POSSIBLE CAUSE
Amenorrhea (absence of menstruation)	Entire Pregnancy	Travel, fatigue, stress, ultra marathoning. She's a He.
Frequent urination	6–8 weeks after conception	She's a woman.
	During car rides	
Food Cravings	First Trimester	You married a fatty.
Fetal movements felt through abdomen	After 16 weeks	Carrying destructive space alien with acid for blood that will burst through stomach lining soon. Bad indigestion.
Delivered child in bathroom during senior prom	9 months	No other cause. But what the hell were you doing marrying a high school senior? You ought to be ashamed.

Pregnancy Tests

Of course, if you want to be sure that your wife is pregnant before she gives birth, the two of you can buy a pregnancy test kit. There are a variety of over-the-counter pregnancy test kits, and each one of them is remarkably accurate. They are also extremely easy to read. Just use this easy chart:

HOW TO READ A PREGNANCY TEST

WHAT THE STICK SHOWS	WHAT IT MEANS
●	Not pregnant.
●●	Pregnant.
	Your wife peed on the Publisher's Clearinghouse form.
|	Not Pregnant.
||	Pregnant.
	Pregnant with a serial killer who plans on murdering people for each of the seven deadly sins. Hopefully, you and your mate are in a traditional, church-sanctioned marriage.
	May be pregnant. May not be. What do you think you see? The conundrum should resolve itself after slightly under a year's worth of therapy.

Sometimes, however, you may suspect that a woman is pregnant and doesn't want to tell you. If this woman is your wife, then you are in serious relationship trouble and you should seek counseling immediately. But you might suspect that a friend is pregnant. Or your sister. Whatever. The important thing is that there are still a few simple tests you can use to determine whether a woman knows she's pregnant. These time-honored techniques are many a man's first source of information:

- Offer to take her to Magic Mountain to ride "The Viper"—a thrilling, steel rollercoaster complete with a 188-foot vertical drop, a top speed approaching 70 mph, and an unprecedented 7 vertical inversions.
- Buy her a round of drinks.
- Ask if she'd like to go off-roading in your sport-utility vehicle.

If a woman won't take you up on any of these offers, then she may be pregnant. Of course, she just may not like really cool, fun things. You'd be surprised how many women don't.

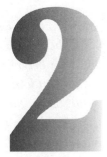

Nine Months
and Counting

She's puking her guts out every morning despite not drinking the night before. She's getting fatter and fatter. And the doctor says she's pregnant.

Congratulations! Your boys can swim!

But, now that you know you're not shooting blanks, you're going to have a whole new set of concerns and questions. Will you be asked to do more around the house? What if the child is actually a devil child, whose birth ushers in the dawn of a dark and evil millennium? Even though neither you nor your wife is Dominican, can you still hope that your child will become the highest-paid utility infielder in the history of sport?

Four

Establishing Paternity

Sure, she's the mother. But are you the father? This may well be your biggest concern throughout your wife's pregnancy.

Unfortunately, women don't have glass stomachs so you can watch the development of the child. That would be really cool, although undoubtedly slightly off-putting. As a result, you don't know exactly when conception occurred. Furthermore, you don't really know whether the child is yours! Without medical testing, you can't determine the paternity of the child until it's born, and even then, newborns all look about the same—all red-faced and yicky.

But establishing paternity is important. Because you certainly don't want to get up in the middle of the night to go get pickles and ice cream just to make sure the postman's kid comes out okay. On the other hand, your wife will get extremely offended if you ask her to take a DNA test. It's a question you can ask only if you have a strong suspicion that the baby is not yours. Use the following checklist to determine whether you should insist on a DNA test.

POSSIBLE SIGNS THE BABY ISN'T YOURS:

- The FedEx guy often comes by with "special deliveries," yet you don't recall ever getting a package.
- You haven't slept with your wife for the past year.
- Your old next-door neighbor hurriedly left town around the time your wife started showing.
- Your wife is jokingly referred to by your poker buddies as "the town slut."
- Your wife invites you to appear on the *Jerry Springer Show*.

Once the baby is born, there are much more obvious signs that the child is not legitimate. Look for the following dead giveaways:

- The Child has a 666 birthmark on its head, and is constantly looked after by a strict German governess and her pair of highly-trained Dobermans.
- The baby turns out half-Tongan. (Note: Disregard if either you or your wife is actually Tongan. However, if both of you are Tongan, pay attention. Also, don't eat too many salty foods, as high blood pressure plagues Pacific Islanders.)
- Three clowns dressed as kings show up at your door bearing frankincense, myrrh, and gold. They say they found your place by following a shining star.

Finances

Having a child is not cheap. You'll need to buy baby food, diapers, toys, and, in Arkansas, guns.

Unfortunately, the projected total cost of putting a single child through a four-year private college in the year 2020 is a whopping 787,000 dollars!!! And the price for twins is approximately double that!!

Conventional investments can't possibly cover that enormous sum. There is, however, a powerful money-making tool designed to raise just this sort of cash in a hurry, and, amazingly enough, without you having to leave your home! The secret??? Mail-order investing!

Just send fifteen dollars cash to the person at the top of the following Big Money List to receive an informative leaflet about mail-order investing.

THE BIG MONEY LIST
Mason Brown
10850 Wilshire Blvd., #1000
Westwood, CA 90025

Martin Brown
10850 Wilshire Blvd., Suite 1000
Westwood, CA 90025

Macon Brown
10850 Wilshire Blvd., Box 1000
Westwood, CA 90025

Maran Brown
10850 Wilshire Blvd., Apt. 1000
Westwood, CA 90025

After you've received your leaflet, remove the top name and
bump everyone up a notch. Put your name at the bottom, and
send the revised list to everyone you know. By the time they've
followed the instructions, you could find yourself the recipient of over one million dollars!!! That's not too shabby for just
fifteen dollars and the price of a few postage stamps.

This scheme is totally legal and is not a "Ponzi" or "pyramid" scheme in any way, shape, or form. Just don't send your
letters to any prosecuting attorneys (they're notoriously
cheap).

Other Ways to Make Money

Of course, there's no need for you to do all the work. What better way to instill the virtues of thrift and industry than by starting your child off in business at an early age? Let him feel the responsibility of pulling his own weight (which, given the exorbitant cost of baby supplies, will be far greater than his listed ten pounds). Forget about lemonade stands, today's child has a plethora of high-paying career options.

Textile Mill Operator: Textile mills, with all their whirring, intricate machinery, always require fresh hands. And a child's slender, nimble fingers are naturally suited to the task. While the hourly wage isn't great, the pay can still be impressive due to the fourteen-hour shifts, seven days a week. And if your child is lucky, who knows? Maybe he'll get a visit from renowned mother Kathie Lee Gifford.

Child Actor: Nobody gets as overpaid as actors do, except sports figures. And nobody (except perhaps fans of women's gymnastics) wants to see toddlers in action. So why not get Junior to follow in the footsteps of such child stars as Gary Coleman, Drew Barrymore, and Dana Plato. And who knows? If the acting doesn't work out, there's always a video store just around the corner.

Organ Donor: The math is simple. A child is born with two kidneys. It only needs one. Yet on the human organ black market, a healthy kidney in perfect condition can go for as much as fifty thousand dollars. One other solid money maker—bone marrow transplants. Sure, these operations are excruciatingly painful, but while an adult remembers pain, infants forget. Ask yourself, can you recall anything that happened to you when you were less than a year old? I can't remember my circumcision but I bet you anything it stung like the dickens.

Choosing (and Working with) Your Practitioner

Your wife will want to choose a top-flight OB-GYN specialist from a world-recognized medical institution. So will you, until you see the price tag. Holy moley!!! These guys make more than plumbers!!

Thankfully, in today's brave new world, women are more and more open to alternative kinds of childbirth providers, many of which are substantially more reasonable pricewise than their so-called "expert" counterparts. Remember, people were delivering children long before the first medical school. How hard can it be? So don't throw your money away on a doctor before you've considered all of your options.

Alternative Childbirth Providers

Taxi Driver: Everyone knows that cabbies make great midwives. Behind that gruff, crusty, cigar-chomping exterior lies the cool calm of a great doctor. If your wife has ever seen lovable Vic Tayback in *The Great American Traffic Jam*, she won't be satisfied by anything less than an authentic Los Angeles livery driver. Interesting hygiene tip: Why boil water when a sweat-stained, white tank top will do just fine?

Rates: Very Competitive. $1.90 to start, then ¢.20 each additional quarter mile or fraction thereof.

Downside: Must name the child after the driver.

Stewardess: You may think of stewardesses as glorified flying waitresses, but these plucky little women are actually angels riding aloft on titanium wings. They can keep a planeload of passengers calm even after the captain has been sucked out of the cockpit in a giant explosion. Imagine how soothing they'll be with your wife.

Rates: Very competitive, especially if you're redeeming your frequent-flyer miles.

Downside: Normally loose stews tend to be frigid with you after they've delivered your child.

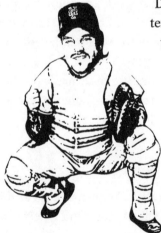

Major League Catcher: If these world-class athletes can catch a hundred-mile-per-hour baseball speeding so fast that it looks like a tiny little pill, then they should have no problem handling a baby moving at a couple of inches per hour. And if the delivery is going poorly, they're not afraid to call time, hold a conference on the mound, and try to talk the woman through it.

Rates: High. Figure at least 2 million for a one year deal.

Downside: May try to renegotiate salary during labor.

Midwives: Since the time of the cavemen, women have shooed men out of the home (although in their case, a cave, presumably) and helped with the delivery. This still goes on today, with midwives as hairy-legged as their predecessors offering birth-at-home assistance.

Rates: Cheaper than doctors by miles.

Downside: There's something pretty dykey about the whole midwife scene, and not in the good "lipstick lesbian" way.

Do-It-Yourself: There's no better way to prove your skill as a handyman than to deliver your own baby. Except, perhaps, by making a particularly well-joined maple sideboard.

Rates: Free. You can't beat that.

Downside: It is sooooo gross.

Traditional OB-GYN

Your wife may insist on a so-called "real" doctor. Fine. But if you're going to shell out that kind of money, then you should make sure you get what you paid for. If your doctor exhibits any of the following signs, then change doctors immediately.

Ways to Tell that Your Wife's Gynecologist Is a Quack

- Uncontrollable laughter whenever he hears the word "vagina."
- Slips off his rubber glove right before any examinations.
- Wears one of those big mirror headbands.
- He makes house calls.
- His medical school diploma has palm trees on the side.

Seven

The Best Odds Diet for Men

T he "Best Odds Diet" for women recommends that pregnant women eat twenty-eight servings of healthy, protein- and vitamin-rich food every day. Twenty-eight servings! Whoa! That's pretty much everything within her reach. The take-home rule: when your wife's eating, keep your hands clear.

Many expectant fathers fall into the trap of eating what their wife eats, and end up gaining weight along with her (known as "Couvade Syndrome," or in layman's terms, "the big, fatty, lard-ass effect"). These men receive several impressive benefits from their increase in size. They are seen as empathic, caring husbands by their wives. They are seen as empathic, caring husbands by their mistresses. And, perhaps most importantly, they are regarded as kings in certain Polynesian island chains, where bulk is directly proportional to spiritual power.

Unfortunately for many would-be Samoan potentates, some American men often have difficulty putting on massive quantities of weight. They can eat and eat and eat and still look like a stick. This can mean big trouble for a marriage, too, since women who are gaining weight invariably become outraged at sticklike men with high metabolisms.

If you are one of these lean men, don't despair. You can put on weight if you know what you're doing. A proper understanding of what is known as the "nutritional pyramid" can help you pack on the empathic pregnancy pounds. With dedication and persistence you'll become so fat you'll at least look like you really love your wife.

The Nutritional Pyramid.

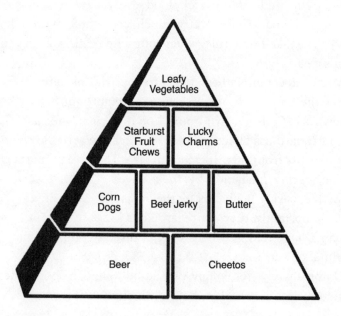

Leafy Vegetables

Starburst Fruit Chews | Lucky Charms

Corn Dogs | Beef Jerky | Butter

Beer | Cheetos

The Nutritional Pyramid Explained

The key to the nutritional pyramid is a full understanding of the principle of "empty" calories. An empty calorie is a calorie without any nutritional value whatsoever, such as you could find in a cheese puff. Your body will turn this calorie into fat immediately. And because your body does actually need some nutrients, you will quickly become hungry again.

LEAFY VEGETABLES:
Packed with vitamins and minerals, and low in calories, these dreaded weeds can overrun the intestines before any quality fat is generated. Eat sparingly—no more than one serving a day. Be exceedingly watchful since vegetables can turn up in food you thought was safe. Burgers, for instance, often have lettuce or tomatoes on them. Consider taking them off before you eat the burger. Be especially wary of dark vegetables such as kale. In fact, if you even know what kale is, you are going to have real problems gaining weight.

STARBURST FRUIT CHEWS:
Not even pregnant Samoans want their husbands to have teeth as bad as the English, so you must make sure your body gets the vitamin C it needs to prevent scurvy. The problem is that real fruit contains fiber, and nothing slows down weight gain like regularity. No, for your purposes, you want one bowel movement every other day, tops. Starburst Fruit Chews provide the ideal compromise. Filled with sugar calories, and 100 percent fiber-free, they are the ideal health food.

Lucky Charms:
Along with important vitamins and minerals (such as A, D, E, K, B1–12, and Iron), your body also needs Pink Hearts, Green Clovers, Yellow Moons, Blue Diamonds and Purple Horseshoes. Oh, and lots of pure sugar. It's a scientific fact.

Corn Dogs:
As revered in the Orient for virility-enhancing powers as powdered rhinoceros horn, and significantly more tasty, corn dogs are an essential part of a balanced diet. As one anonymous wag/dietitian noted, "Corn dogs put the 'nut' in nutrition."

Beef Jerky:
It's vital to have some food around the house that only you like. If you don't, your wife will eat it all and you will be left with nothing. Fortunately, pregnant women rarely find spicy, greasy sticks of flavored beef lard appealing. That's why it's vital that you have a supply of cured beef strips in your cupboard. You need food, too! And jerky, despite it's tough texture, is one of the most effective weight gainers in the world. So snap into a Slim Jim, and step into fitness.

Butter:
Men like butter. Get sticks and sticks of it. Don't just use it on toast or muffins, smear it on everything except your wife (now's not the time to play Marlon Brando in *Last Tango in Paris*).

Beer:

Ah, Beer. Hailed by the ancient Sumerians as the nectar of the Gods, or at least as a nice way of getting drunk, beer is truly a staple of fathers around the world. First of all, it's alcoholic, so Mom's not allowed to dip into your supply. Second, beer allows you to "think outside of the box" when looking for solutions to difficult problems. For instance, when confronted with the brutal cost of sending a child through college, very few child-rearing books even mention the money that a drug courier (or "mule") can make in just one trip back from Colombia. Yet after only a couple of beers, you might come up with the idea of making your child ingest condoms filled with cocaine. Problem solved. Just beware—too many beers and you may find yourself thinking "inside the bowl."

Cheetos:

"Cheetos" includes all of the chip sub-groups—Doritos, Fritos, Pretzels, Beer Nuts, Nachos, and Funyons. These so-called "designer super foods" aren't just for snacking anymore. Make sure you include at least one large bag at each meal, and you'll be fatter than your wife in no time. And once that glorious day arrives, you'll be able to say "we're pregnant" without a trace of irony. Congratulations.

Your Wife's Nutritional Needs

Your wife will be getting all sorts of advice about how to eat healthily. In her desire to make sure the baby develops properly, the odds are she will take all of it. Turn her maternal instinct to your advantage—stress that science proves that pregnant women need much more protein in their diet than nonpregnant women. Mention that sperm is an ideal source of fat-free protein. Recommend that she have at least one serving daily.

Eight

Prenatal Care 101

O bviously, the most important prenatal care duties belong to the mother. After all, she is the incubator for your soon-to-be baby. Do not, however, refer to your wife as "the incubator" while she's within earshot.

But prenatal care is not just a mother's burden. Fathers also play an important role that ensures proper prenatal care. You have two vital jobs to perform—making sure that you yourself don't do anything stupid to harm the baby, and making sure that the mother doesn't unknowingly do something harmful.

Regulating Your Own Behavior

Making sure you don't do anything that's harmful to the baby sounds easy, but it isn't. Just take a look at all the things you've got to give up:

- No smoking: You don't want the baby to be a victim of secondhand smoke inhalation.

- No smoking dope: See above.
- No throwing the medicine ball around with the wife.
- No couples weekends at Six Flags in Sandusky, Ohio, even if it is the home of "G-Force: the Ride!"
- No sharing needles.
- No "punch me in the stomach hard" contests with the wife.
- No waking up in the middle of the night screaming "I'll kill you all, you Charlie bastards!"
- No group sex.
- No tag team sit-up marathons.
- No tandem assault on Everest.

The list goes on and on. There's no end to your sacrifices. I mean, sure, you could summit Everest solo, but that's only half as fun. Besides, with the time constraints such a climb demands, you could really hurt a marriage by being away for so long. So if you want to stay together, you'll have to wait until you can at least put the baby in one of those Swedish papoose knapsacks before heading into thin air as a family.

Regulating Your Wife's Behavior

Regulating your wife's behavior is much more satisfying. Have you ever wished you could get back at your wife for all the times she's nagged you? Well, now is your chance. Given modern science's ever-increasing knowledge about prenatal care, your wife will do something that's bad for the baby every day. Let her know about her error, no matter how small. Really lay into her. You're just doing it for the good of the baby. Besides, you'll never have another opportunity to criticize her daily and get away with it.

The following table shows some common errors your wife might make, and some sample responses that are appropriate to each mishap:

If you continuously reprimand your wife sharply for each

HER BEHAVIOR	YOUR RESPONSE
She drinks a cup of coffee.	Jesus, Lord!! Think of the baby!!! Are you trying to kill my unborn child??"
She picks the Sunday paper up off the front lawn.	"No, God! Noooooo!!"
She sleeps on her back.	Violently shake her awake. Scream, "You're cutting off the blood supply to the placenta!!! We can only pray the baby will live!!" Then return to sleep.

mistake she makes during the prenatal period, you should reap one very important benefit. Your wife will stop asking you to read child-care books, fearing that any further information you might discover will subsequently be used against her. If you're exceptionally persistent, she might even ask that you not go to breathing class with her. If so, congratulations! You have avoided one of the world's great horrors (see Chapter Seventeen).

Your wife may also develop a nervous condition, causing her to break down and cry at random intervals. Don't worry. It's just hormones. Keep up the steady stream of verbal abuse.

Nine

Sex During Pregnancy

O ne of the most important concerns a man has during pregnancy is what the ramifications will be on his sex life. This is a valid concern because things will be different. Your wife's sex drive may increase or decrease. Your own sex drive may change. You won't want to do anything that might injure the baby with your massive unit. There are a whole host of issues.

Making Her Feel Attractive

The most important thing to do to ensure a healthy sex life during pregnancy is to make sure your wife knows that you still find her body sexually attractive. It's hard for women to feel sexually aroused unless they feel like they look sexy. This is in direct contrast to men, who can pop a woody while farting cabbage gas.

There are many different ways to convince your wife that you still find her desirable—through verbal reassurances, repeated gentle caresses, leaving "specialty" pregnancy fetish magazines lying around the house, etc. One great way to show your appreciation of the pregnant female form is to get a pair of silver mudflaps for your car.

Sexual Positions

Pregnancy does involve very real changes to the female form. Previously favorite coital positions may become uncomfortable or downright impossible. The most obvious example is the "missionary" (man-on-top) position. Simple physics dictates that this position cannot work anymore. A very pregnant woman's belly will have expanded too much. Other positions may also become unpleasant. "Woman-on-top," for instance, suffers considerably upon the addition of twenty to thirty pounds. And any kind of "pleasure swing" apparatus is right out.

That does not mean that you cannot have sex. Far from it! You might even find that your sex life improves now that you don't have to worry about unwanted pregnancy. The following positions, taken from Mason Brown's *Pregnancy Pillow Book*, illustrate some of the exciting possibilities that are still open to the pregnant couple:

- Spooning: This position occurs when the man and woman are on their sides, with the man gently penetrating his partner from behind, supposedly reminiscent of spoons in a drawer—although this author rarely thinks of his cutlery in such graphically sexual terms. If he did, he would never be able to eat soup.

- Solo: The easiest of positions to get into; the man withdraws to the bathroom or bedroom with certain reading material. Considerate partners will hang a "do not disturb" sign in order to minimize unpleasant shock to their spouses.

- The Sphere of a Thousand Loves: This position requires that both partners strap themselves together onto a Gyrosphere and spin themselves into Zero-G ecstasy.*

Oral Sex

During pregnancy, just like in the White House, oral sex is always permissible, at least insofar as the man is the recipient. There are very few occasions (such as when a woman has been judged at high risk of going into labor prematurely) that a female orgasm is not recommended. For those of you who would like to avoid any reciprocation, however, feel free to yell, "Think of the baby!"

If your wife is reluctant to perform oral sex to completion, inform her that according to the July 1998 issue of *Low Country Girl* magazine, Dutch researchers have reported that semen ingestion may prevent preeclampsia. Do NOT inform her

---

*Caution!! The effects of the Gyrosphere on fetal development have not been researched, quite possibly because it is so blatantly dangerous.

that this same study also found that sex with Dutch re-searchers promoted "an overall sense of well-being to good-looking women everywhere."

Sex with Strangers

Many sexologists recommend multiple anonymous partners throughout life, and pregnancy is no exception. The fact that they make a living as sexologists should lead you to consider their findings with caution, however. While some of them may indeed be experts, they are all, at the very least, super-horny experts.

More reliable counselors stick to the following rule: Sleeping with strangers should absolutely be avoided. That is not to say that sleeping with acquaintances or friends is permitted. No, no. That is completely out, too. Strictly *verboten*. Really, I shouldn't even have to tell you all this.

Frequently Asked Questions about Sex and Pregnancy

My wife loves to kiss me as soon as she wakes up. I used to think it was cute, but now she gets sick in the morning and she still wants a kiss!!!! What should I do?

Tell her, "No way, you stinking puke breath!" That way she'll understand your reluctance.

I love engaging in unprotected anal intercourse with Haitian she-male hookers, but I worry about the possibility of catching a yicky disease like crabs. Of course, I shave my scrotum, so I should be able to see the little buggers if they're there.

Sounds like you should be okay.

My wife's sex drive has gotten really high since she got pregnant. I'm having trouble keeping up. What should I do?

First of all, stop whining! Next, eat some eggs and tuna fish while reading graphic pornography. Problem solved.

I worry that I might hurt the baby when I make love to my wife. Can I?

I don't know. How big is your nob? If it's smaller than average (ten inches or less), probably not.

My wife doesn't seem to want to have sex with me now that she's pregnant. How can I change this?

Get a better job and surround yourself with good-looking, highly sexual personal secretaries. She'll come around fast. And if she doesn't, what's it to you?

Ten

What's Going On in There?

Understanding the Trimester System

Women will look at you in horror if you tell them that your four-month pregnant wife is in her first semester. Yet college-educated men often stumble over the correct terminology. Familiar as they are with semesters (or, in State Colleges, quarters), trimesters come as a complete surprise.

Gaffes such as these can be avoided with a cursory examination of the process of fetal development.

The First Trimester

Insemination: Your sperm swam to her egg. This was not as easy as it sounds. The following diagram illustrates the perils of a sperm's journey.

From the moment of conception, the embryo starts dividing and redividing at an incredibly rapid pace. Yet for the first three months it is virtually impossible to differentiate the embryo from that of other animals. Indeed, scientists once postulated

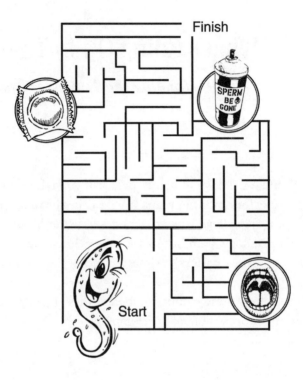

that the embryo had to pass through all prior phases of evolution on the way to becoming human, from fish to primate. Of course, these scientists were insane, Moreau-like men, complete with dwarf helpers. Nonetheless, this startling photo of a two-month-old fetus may explain their belief. It may also explain their seemingly irrational belief that the womb environment resembled postwar Tokyo. The fetus, however, unlike the king of Monster Island, cannot survive outside its mother at this age.

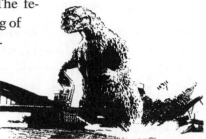

The Second Trimester

The fetus at two months

The second trimester includes months four, five, and six. During this time, the fetus starts to look human and begins to develop its sense of taste, presumably much to its dismay as it is completely immersed in a combination of amniotic fluid and its own urine. Certain decadent Germans, however, never outgrow a craving for this taste.

The fetus begins kicking and performing somersaults during this time. Its heart will be clearly audible using a hand held ultrasound device called a Doppler. Its pulse rate of 140-beats-per-minute will stun even the most out-of-shape father-to-be. Don't panic. It's supposed to sound like a marching band on crank. As the fetus grows, its kicks will become stronger. If you're lucky, you may get to feel one through your wife's abdomen. Ultrasound pictures clearly show how much force a developing fetus can generate.

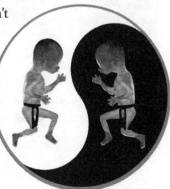

The Third Trimester

The last three months of pregnancy are an important time for the fetus. They are a period of great growth, especially of the brain. Some experts recommend that the mother listen to classical music during this time, to stimulate neural connections. The disparity between those who listen to Mozart and those who listen to nothing is apparent in the following ultrasound images.

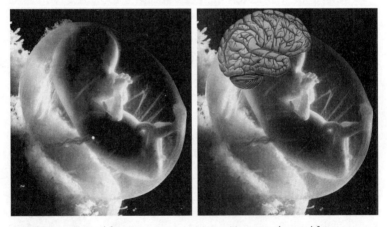

Normal fetus   Mozart-enhanced fetus

Although the far-superior brain capacity of the acoustically stimulated infant is obviously preferable, be careful. Too much classical music, especially Wagner, can actually lead to complications during delivery.

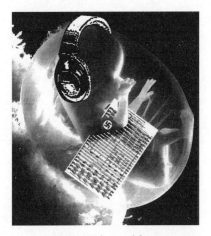

Wagner-enhanced fetus

Similarly, obstetricians everywhere agree that it is vital that mothers of twins NEVER watch the *Jerry Springer Show*.

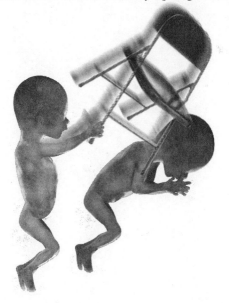

Your Wife's Mental Changes Throughout Pregnancy

Y ou must understand that not only does your wife's body change throughout pregnancy, but so too does her mental state. With each passing month, your wife must mentally adjust to her new hormones and body shape. Fatigue will come easier, as will sudden mood changes. She may feel an increase in sexual desire, or a decrease. Flatulence will almost certainly become a problem. Beware! Once a woman realizes she can fart without repercussions, her entire outlook on life changes. The heady rush of freedom each gassy expulsion provides sends many pregnant women down the path of lesbianism and into the murky world of women's golf. That's a proven scientific fact, not just idle conjecture.

A recent study asked men to keep a chart of what they felt their wife's mental state to be throughout pregnancy. The results were fascinating.

	PRE-PREGNANCY	FIRST TRIMESTER	SECOND TRIMESTER	THIRD TRIMESTER	POST-PARTUM
HUSBANDS' DESCRIPTIONS OF THEIR WIVES' MENTAL STATE THROUGHOUT PREGNANCY					
Husband 1	Sweetness and laughter.	Moody and anxious.	Joy and excitement.	Anticipation. Eagerness.	Relieved, yet slightly sad.
Husband 2	Cranky and irritating.	Cranky and irritating.	Cranky and irritating.	Cranky and irritating.	Cranky and irritating.
Husband 3	Endearingly quirky.	Elation.	Manic energy. Constant cleaning.	Irregular outbursts of laughter at odd times of the night.	She drove the twins into a goddamn lake!!

Significantly, this study, with its sample pool of only three men, has little or no statistical merit. But as anecdotal evidence, it's pretty powerful stuff.

Coping Strategies

Your wife will experience a whole range of emotions during her pregnancy, and you will bear the brunt of these wild mood swings. You must have specific coping strategies planned out for each of her moods, or you will be completely over-whelmed, saucer-eyed and helpless. Don't think you can rely on your natural instincts. As the following table illustrates, your natural response is often the exact opposite of the correct response.

POSSIBLE SIGNS THAT YOUR WIFE IS PREGNANT

HER EMOTIONAL STATE	YOUR NATURAL RESPONSE	THE CORRECT RESPONSE
Fatigue	To help with the household chores.	Don't be an enabler! Make her get up and work or she risks becoming codependent for life!
Joy	To smile with her.	Avoid her. Joy is soon followed by anger due to some moronic thing you've done.
Anger	To talk things through and resolve matters lovingly.	Flee! The anger of a pregnant woman is exponentially compounded because she realizes that her potentially perfect child will be ruined by your hopelessly flawed genes.

Twelve

The Working Mother

I n today's society, many couples find that both partners work. And so, many women wonder how many months into the pregnancy they should work before taking time off.

Thanks to modern technologies such as the laptop PC and the cell phone, the answer has never been easier: nine. In fact, women can work straight through pregnancy. Typically, contractions during active labor are one minute long with three- to five-minute intervals between them. Well, you're not an ogre. You don't expect your wife to work while she's having contractions. But what about the rest intervals? Hello-ooo?? Up and at 'em, lazy bones!

And with a properly applied epidural, there doesn't have to be any downtime at all. She should be able to hammer out PowerPoint presentations right up until the time comes to push.

But don't think her earning potential ends there. Far from it. Hook up a digital video camera and broadcast the miracle of birth over the Internet. You'd be surprised how much money you can make selling the live feed to fans of the "specialty" genre by using the Adult Vericheck system. To stave off any possible prosecution, remember to "mirror" your website to an Amsterdam URL (where there are seemingly no laws whatsoever).

The earnings don't stop there, either. After your baby starts suckling, your wife's milk should come in. Don't waste a precious drop! Hook her up to a breast pump immediately, and she can hold two jobs easily—her current one, as well as wet nurse. And don't forget to maintain your website's video feed. People will pay good money to see her lactate. If she feels up to it (and why wouldn't she), add a chat room for VIP members. Who knew pregnancy could be this profitable?

Thirteen

The Gender Dilemma

Should You Find Out the Sex
of Your Unborn Child?

At three months, your doctor will perform an ultrasound exam that can reveal the sex of your unborn child. Some Luddite couples prefer not to be told the results of this test, preferring instead to retain the element of surprise by smashing the ultrasound machine to pieces with a sledgehammer. Other parents cannot avoid finding out, as the doctor cries out, "My God! Look at the size of that thing! I'm getting out of here before it goes off!"

Most parents, however, do request to be informed of the baby's gender. And rightfully so. They are still surprised when they find out the baby's sex, they just find out earlier—in time to make good money on the office pool. These couples can also get started right away on important tasks such as decorating the child's room, buying clothes for the baby, and, if it's a girl and you are reading the Chinese translation of this book, selling her off to the highest bidder. In fact, as any reputable child-care book will tell you, couples who decide not to be told are big losers who invariably make bad parents.

Assuming you decide to find out, you must be careful not to let your wife know that you have a preference. She'll pretend not to care, even though she wants a girl to play dress-up with. You should feign nonchalance as well. It will be a little game you play, despite the fact that, obviously, you want a boy. For one thing, a boy will carry on the family name (although in my personal experience it seems unlikely that the name "Brown" will die out).

Half the time you won't get what you want. Yet you must look on the bright side. While you may think that all women are monstrous creatures with toothed vaginas lying in wait to devour the unwary, that's just not the case. In fact, that's pretty damn neurotic and you should seek help.

The following table demonstrates the pros and cons of having a boy or a girl. You may be surprised at its conclusion.

BOYS VS. GIRLS

BOYS	GIRLS

ATHLETICS

Fun to play catch with.

Edge: Boys

Throw like girls.

HOMEWORK

Will ask smart school chum for "help" on hard, take-home math tests.

Edge: Boys

Will ask you for help on hard, take-home math tests.

CLOTHES

Will borrow your clothes to appear retro, making you feel like an old dork.

Will borrow Mom's clothes to appear retro, making her feel like an old dork.

Edge: Girls

HIGH SCHOOL YEARS

May vow revenge against all the snooty girls in class, then take gun to school and go on killing spree

     Edge: Draw

May be a snooty girl

COLLEGE YEARS

Will drink too much, experiment with drugs, and prove a great overall disappointment. During summers, his fraternity brothers will "crash" at your place.

Will drink too much, experiment with drugs, and prove a great overall disappointment. During summers, her sorority sisters will "crash" at your place.

Edge: Girls

AND THE WINNER IS: Girls!! Whenever twenty-one-year-old coeds use your house to host a sorority slumber party, you can die a happy man. Which is good, because as soon as your wife realizes what's going on in your head, she will kill you.

Fourteen

Naming Your Baby

Don't kid yourself. If you choose a stupid name for your baby, he will hate you forever. He will curse your name and spit on your grave. He will have you exhumed, then mount your body in a display case where you are perpetually ass-raped by an animatronic polar bear.

And he'll be right to do so. Especially if you give him some pansy name like Dakota.

Some of you will be tempted to follow the old Native American tradition of naming your child after the first thing you see after he's born. Don't fall into this trap. Because while this system may work well in the wild outdoors (Running Bear, Sitting Bull, Chief Knockahoma, etc.), it does not work in the confines of the modern hospital. Step outside the delivery room of any modern, urban hospital and you will come up with names like: Annoying Guy on Cell Phone, Shuffling Crazy Guy, Smelly Janitor, Irvin the Slightly Befuddled Resident on a New Rotation, or Filipino Nurse in a Hurry. While these names are unusual, they also suck ass.

Family Names

Of course, the old standby way of naming babies is to just name the child after an ancestor. The obvious problem with this method is that just two generations ago, people had incredibly stupid names like Dolores or Dwight. And if you look back even further, you're talking about Civil War–era names like Euphemia or Ulysses. Remember that these were people who thought that muttonchop sideburns were cool.

Worse yet, as an American, there's a better than fifty-fifty chance that you come from immigrant stock. God forbid you use an old-country name like Shlomo. You'll doom your child to a life in the garment district (or whatever stereotypical occupation your particular ethnic group may happen to be cursed with). WASPs may think they're exempt from this warning, but name a child Nigel and just see if he doesn't turn out to enjoy gobbling nob in an anonymous glory hole near the theater district.

Biblical Names

All too often, our ancestors chose Old Testament biblical names and, trust me, today's child would rather get tossed into an overheated oven than spend a minute in a playground with a name like Shadrach, Meshach, or Abednego. Not only that, biblical names tend to run a little on the long side. You try and fill in Nebuchadnezzar in the space provided in your SAT booklet. It's a nightmare.

As for New Testament names, your choices are limited. If you like Matthew, Mark, Luke, or John, go right ahead. Paul, Timothy, and Andrew are fine, too. But, please, pass on Titus.

Baby Name Books

Many couples buy a book with lists of popular baby names. These books are readily obtainable at the checkout counter of any reputable twenty-four-hour drugstore. While these lists are acceptable in and of themselves, using such a list unfortunately means that your child may be branded as a baby whose parents use all-night pharmacies.

All baby name books break down names by sex. This is fine. However, names give us much more information than just gender. For instance, if your parents called you "Enis Bratlovski," then there's no way in hell anybody will ever call you "Mr. President." If you name your daughter Brittani, then you shouldn't complain when she turns out to be a stripper. And how many white women are named Tamika?

The following is a list of boys' and girls' names, followed by what the names mean in their original language, as well as what they mean today.

BOYS' NAMES

NAME	LANGUAGE	ORIGINAL MEANING	TODAY'S MEANING
Leo	Latin	Lion	Somebody liked *Titanic* a little too much.
Antawn	Ebonics	"Worthy of Praise."	My parents can't spell.
Wendell	Teutonic	A Wend (a Slavic people living between the Elbe and the Ober).	Kick me now!
Kang	Klingon	Nothing. It's a stupid, made-up language.	My parents are Trekkies. Somebody please help me.
Jack	Irish	Variant of John, Hebrew for "God is merciful."	My parents used a focus group to come up with a name.
Mason	English	Stoneworker.	Great author and magnificent lover.
Conan	Scottish	Knowledgeable.	Weenie talk show host; Man who lives on Funyons.
Pablo	Spanish	Small.	Man with huge testicles and overrated drawing skills.
Jesus	Hebrew	Son of God.	Utility infielder from the Dominican Republic.
Chaim	Hebrew	To Life.	I'm a Jew.
Adolf	German	Wolf.	When I grow up, I'm going to be a guest on *Jerry Springer*.
Benito	Italian	Blessed.	At least, I'm not named Adolf.

GIRLS' NAMES

NAME	LANGUAGE	ORIGINAL MEANING	TODAY'S MEANING
Candi	Latin	From Candace. Fire, White, Pure, Glowing.	Stripper.
Vikki	Latin	Victory.	Jell-O wrestler.
Divine	English	Divine.	Black hooker.
Nikki	Greek	Victory of the People.	White hooker.
Holly	English	Plant with red berries.	Body-to-body masseuse, complete with happy ending.
Doreen	Irish	Sullen.	Nevada state-licensed prostitute.
Tiffany	Greek	Manifestation of God.	Call girl.
Mistress Greta	Greek	From Margaret. A Pearl.	Dominatrix.

The astute reader will note that no one ever names their daughter "Mistress" anything. Well, name your daughter Greta and you might as well buy her a whip and a red rubber ball gag for the baby shower.

Fifteen

The Baby Shower

Once your wife is more than three months into her pregnancy, she'll want to start planning her baby shower. That's fine. Encourage her. It will keep her occupied for weeks. Do NOT get suckered in to helping her!! This is a role reserved for her best friend or sister. Just as the best man prepares the bachelor party, so too should the maid of honor* prepare the baby shower.

Your wife will ask you if you want the baby shower to be coed. The answer is no. No. No. No. A thousand times, no. Your male friends will never forgive you if you trap them into attending a baby shower. Stories abound of men gathering the ribbons of the baby presents, pretending they're going to play

---

* If the maid of honor and your wife are no longer speaking for whatever reason (like, say, she reveals to your wife that you recently banged her in a closet at a party while you were both wasted), the role devolves to her current equivalent. This probably means the bridesmaid who was next in line. Unless you banged her, too, you scoundrel.

a party game, and then suspending the father-to-be from his testicles on a nearby avocado tree.

Why are baby showers so horrifying? Because it is a time during which women are in control. Emotions are shared, feelings expressed, garden outfits worn. And this brief glimpse of Bizarro World has been enough to turn many a husband into a gibbering idiot, more monkey than man.

And worse yet, this gathering of women is focusing on the source of their power—their ability to nurture life. They will alternately lord this power over you and whip you with guilt, since *they* are going to undergo hideous pain just for you and the baby. They will never relinquish this guilt power, and your wife will abuse it badly the first time she realizes she has it. Especially when the other women egg her on.

Indeed, by the end of a baby shower, the festivities will not resemble a

---

SHOWER GIFTS

While your number one priority is to get out of the house, a distant second is to make sure the baby shower doesn't rake in exclusively boring gifts like clothes and car seats and diaper genies. Sure, those are useful presents, but they're absolutely no fun for you to play with.

The solution? Register at SportMart. You know you kicked yourself for not doing that for wedding presents. Don't make the same error twice. Tell your friends, tell your relatives: The baby needs sporting goods. It's never too early to start molding a champion. Just ask Se Ri Pak's dad. You'll need golf clubs, balls, gloves, and a sleeping bag and tent for camping trips to the local cemetery.

Oh, and the baby could probably use some power tools, too. They're very educational.

And nothing offers more in the way of learning opportunities than a satellite dish with all the premium channels included.

ladies' tea party so much as a witches' coven. The women will play "party games" such as "The Why We Hate Men Game," or "The Power of Platonic Lesbianism Game" or "Gaia, the Earth Mother Song." It's a wonder softball games don't break out (probably because most yards are too small, and no one brings gloves).

Sixteen

Preparing the Baby's Room

S ometime toward the middle of her pregnancy, your wife will want you to prepare the baby's room. She will almost certainly reject your arguments that you paint the interior of the garage blue and toss the crib in there. Any attempts to convert the doghouse into a "babyhouse" are equally doomed.

And since the guest room is reserved for guests, you undoubtedly will have to turn your prized home office into baby central. There go your late nights "working" at home, surfing the Internet for "research." After all, for most people, looking at hardcore lesbian pony-play videos quickly loses its appeal when their newborn child howls in the background. Of course, that's only most people. Some people find the wails of a hungry baby to be an erotic accompaniment that enhances their sexual pleasure immeasurably. These people usually end up in prison.

Assuming you decide to furnish Baby's room instead of

leaving it as your office, there are two schools of thought on how to go about doing so.

The Traditional Plan

Traditional baby room design calls for a soft blue, pink, or yellow pastel paint job, depending on whether your baby is a boy, a girl, or a hermaphrodite. The crib, with regulation one-and-a-quarter-inch space bars, prevents Baby from trapping his head between the bars. Age appropriate toys, such as mirrors and hard rattles, line the room. The baby is constantly monitored via a two-way intercom.

PROS

- Compliance to your wife's wishes will buy you a ten-minute respite before normal fighting resumes.
- When you talk into the intercom, you can pretend you're Captain Kirk. Sure it's geeky, but it's actually kind of fun. Try saying "Spock!" just to get the hang of it.
- It's fun to play with all the cool toys before the baby gets his grubby mitts all over them.

CONS

- Cuteness overload can induce nausea.
- "Cute" truck wallpaper may cause Baby to grow up thinking that long-distance hauling is actually a desirable career choice.
- The "It's a Small World" mobile may lull your child to

sleep, but it may also turn you into an axe-wielding murderer. Use it sparingly.
- The intercom interferes with your sleeping schedule.
- Bo-ring!

The Postmodern Plan

Why saddle yourself with yesteryear's dated notion of child-rearing? Use today's exciting technology to create your own brave new baby. The postmodern baby's room relies on clean architectural steel to instill the aesthetic of the new in your child, and ready him for the cities of tomorrow. Modeled after Jeremy Bentham's revolutionary "Panopticon" penitentiary, two-way mirrors allow you to monitor the baby's movements at all times. When combined with the recommended PA system, you will appear God-like as you scold him for infractions committed when he doesn't think you can possibly see him.

PROS
- Soundproof tiling filters out annoying "crying."
- Stainless-steel floors and walls allow for easy clean up.
- Baby-size hamster wheel lets Baby crawl for miles without getting into trouble.
- A constant barrage from twelve video monitors, evenly spaced around the round room, will allow Baby to speak eight languages by the time he's three. He'll also be well briefed in world financial markets, as well as pop culture.

One possible negative side effect—as an adult, he may wish to grow a Wolf Blitzer beard.

- Painful electrical shocks delivered to the baby at random intervals will quickly induce a Zen-like state of "learned helplessness."
- A wall-mounted feeding tube delivers food at times regulated for your convenience. Baby will adjust to your schedule, or go hungry. The lever-activated treadle option can make eating an educational experience as well.
- Flash-bang grenades make wakey-wakey quick and easy.

CONS

- You're branded a madman.
- Flashing strobe lights can induce seizures.
- Your child will insist that when you reach your thirtieth birthday you go to "Carousel" for recycling. Fail to do so, and you become a "Runner."

Seventeen

Birthing Classes

A t around her seventh or eighth month, your wife will insist that you attend some form of birthing class. This may seem a little irrelevant, since you already know what you need to know—she's going to deliver the baby while you stand around helplessly. Nonetheless, your wife will insist you attend the class with her.

Picking the Class

No matter what class you choose, you will hate it. So, either pick the cheapest class or pick Lamaze. The advantage to picking Lamaze is that you can say, "Oh, we're taking a Lamaze class," and people won't ask you to explain what you're learning or how it differs from Lamaze. The advantage to picking the cheapest class? It's cheaper, you moron!

What You'll Learn

All classes that start off with a group of people in a circle introducing themselves in order invariably turn out to be worthless. Birthing class is no different. In fact, it's worse, since in many small seminars you can at least find out the names and interests of the hot chicks in your class. Here, there are only pregnant women, and they can see that your wife is with you—as can their burly, mustachioed husbands.

THE VIDEO

The first thing your teacher will do is show you a "miracle of life" video. You may hope that the video will focus on the joys of conception and feature attractive Swedish models. You may even associate the warning "graphic details" with positive memories learned in the privacy of your own home in front of your VCR.

Well, too bad! The video shows *delivery* in graphic detail, not conception. There's more blood here than in any Brian De Palma movie ever made. It makes the first thirty minutes of *Saving Private Ryan* look like *Beaches* (although, in this author's opinion, *Beaches* could have been considerably improved if Bette Midler had spent less time yapping and more time looking for her severed arm).

BREATHING

During your classes, you and your spouse will practice taking short, sharp breaths that sound something like this: "Ha ha ha, hee hee hee, ha ha ha." If only your wife made that much noise during sex (although not necessarily those exact sounds).

You will also practice taking deep, cleansing breaths to better cope with the agonizing pain of labor. Why is unclear. When the actual moment comes, she will take an epidural and breathe normally. And, so long as you stand clear of your wife's wildly swinging claw-like hands before the anesthetic takes, you should experience no discomfort at all during labor.

Remember to wear comfortable footgear, however. Should your wife's labor take a long time, you may have to be on your feet for well over ten hours while she's lying down in bed. Without properly fitting sneakers, your dogs will be barking!

BREAST-FEEDING

Birthing class instructors differ on many points. Some think women should walk around during labor, others think they should give birth in a swimming pool (which is extremely thoughtless to the other swimmers, especially those doing laps). But all agree on one point—your wife must breast-feed!

To be sure, it sounds good in theory. Breast milk is free, formula isn't (at least after the first few weeks when they're trying to hook you). Breast-feeding passes the mother's immunities on to the baby (saving on expensive pediatric visits). And it naturally gives the child a boost of up to ten IQ points (worth an estimated five dollars per hour to five hundred thousand dollars per year, depending on your child's base IQ level) without having to spend any extra money on expensive books, and eliminating the tedious task of actually reading them to the child.

But before you go to the dog track with your savings, consider the downside. Your wife's breasts can now squirt milk. Ewwwwwwwwwwwwwwwwwwww!!!

Some men will argue, "Yes, but her breasts are much bigger when she's breast-feeding." Well, your testicles can swell up real big, too, if you get kicked in the balls, but that doesn't mean you want it to happen. Sure, big breasts are a wonderful thing—if you get to play with them. But if you should decide to kiss your wife's lactating breasts in a moment of passion, one of two things will occur. 1) She will say, "Please don't. My nipples are sore." Or 2) you will get a mouthful of nondairy creamer.

One final word of caution. If your wife does decide to breast-feed, do NOT make loud mooing noises while she's doing it. She's much quicker now than she was while pregnant.

Eighteen

What to Bring to the Hospital

A s the delivery date draws closer, it's important that you pack a bag so that you can leave quickly. It's also important that you pack a bag so that you can go to the hospital with your wife should you decide to stay with her and help rear the child.

THE BASIC OVERNIGHT BAG
- Cash

THE RECOMMENDED OVERNIGHT BAG
- Toothbrush
- Toothpaste
- Condoms (Hey, it's not called a "layette" for nothing. Some of those nurses are pretty sexy!)
- Cigars
- Razor scooter (Perfect for long, smooth, linoleum floors; not-so-perfect for maintaining the illusion that you're still "happening.")

- Videotapes: *Alien, Dorf on Golf, Where the Boys Aren't 4*
- *Rolling Stone* magazine (or any other very large magazine. *Life* perhaps).
- *Penthouse Forum* (or any other small collection of pornographic letters and photography that can easily be hidden behind a larger magazine).
- Hand held electronic football game
- Earplugs
- Flask
- A rear-facing baby seat (Do NOT tell them that you drive a two-seater sports car with a passenger side airbag. Some things can be your little secret.)
- An "I'm with stupid" T-shirt and sweatpants for Baby
- An "I'm Stupid" T-shirt and sweatpants for Mommy (She might be angry when she recovers fully from medication. But she'll laugh with you later when she sees the precious pictures of Baby's first days.)
- Five hundred state lotto scratchers (Might as well start planning for your child's future today.)

THE COMPLETE OVERNIGHT BAG
- Everything included in the recommended overnight bag
- Ten thousand dollars in gold bullion (preferably Krugerands)
- Five blank passports of varying nationalities
- His and Her fake mustaches
- Two Glocks with four hundred rounds of ammunition apiece

- One K-Bar survival/combat knife
- Night vision goggles
- GPS Unit
- Compass
- Five-days' worth of bottled water
- Five-days' worth of mixed rations
- Two bars of Toblerone chocolates
- AM/FM/Shortwave radio
- Batteries
- Snakebite kit
- Inflatable raft
- Three Mylar blankets
- Shovel
- Spork (Consider a runcible spoon if a spork is unavailable.)
- His, Her, and Baby's camouflage BDU's
- Five cartons of American cigarettes, for barter use only
- Two bottles of Dewar's scotch whiskey, for medicinal use only
- Two pair nylon stockings, for barter use only (In case you're caught in a space/time flux field and transported back to East Germany, 1946.)
- One French maid's outfit (To help you and your wife perform your duty to humanity and repopulate the earth, if it should come to that.)

These kits should cover every eventuality. Feel free, though, to personalize the kits as you see fit. Try to include your wife in the process. Allow her to pick one item to bring to the hospital. Don't fret, it probably won't weigh you down too much, and if it does, you can always toss it out late at night after you declare the packing complete and she goes to bed.

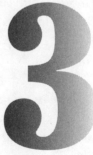

D-Day!!
Labor and Delivery

Most men are caught unawares when the delivery day finally comes around. Why is unclear.

All but the deeply retarded understand that the process takes approximately nine months. Nor were you lacking in physical clues, as your wife grew large enough that it was unsafe for her to go outside in high winds lest she crush unwary pedestrians like a Macy's Day Parade balloon run amok.

Nonetheless, the odds are that you too will shout: "OMyGosh HowCouldThisBeHappeningSoSoonI'mNotReadyIt'sImpossible I'mStillAYoungManDespiteYourObviousAgeWhichIsWhyThe BabyWillBeBornWithHorribleDefectsAndNotDueToMyConstant UsageOfLSDInCollegeWhichWasALongTimeAgoDespiteTheFact ThatI'mStillYoungAndWhatDoYouMeanYou'reInLaborGodHelp UsAll!!!

But don't panic.

Like all gruesome ordeals, such as storming the beaches of Normandy or attending a second cousin's wedding in Atlantic City, the more you shuffle through the event like a mindless zombie, the easier it will be. Familiarize yourself with the step-by-step plan of action set out in the following pages, then try to detach yourself from your body and become a third-party observer. You will perform wonderfully.

Nineteen

Making the Decision to Go to the Hospital

T he first stage of delivery is the onset of labor. Sometimes, however, women experience contractions before they are dilated enough to make a trip to the hospital worthwhile. Since you don't want to waste your valuable television-watching time driving back and forth to the delivery room, you should use this handy table to determine whether your wife is in real labor or whether you can go back to your programs.

DETERMINING WHETHER YOUR WIFE IS IN "REAL" OR "FALSE" LABOR

SIGNS THAT YOUR WIFE IS IN REAL LABOR	SIGNS THAT YOUR WIFE IS IN FALSE LABOR
Her mucus plug hits you in the head from across the room.	Rule #1: She's not in real labor until the game is over, no matter what's happening.
She begs you to drive her to the hospital.	She wants you to stop for ice cream on the way.
Her contractions are coming regularly at three- to five-minute intervals	You are squeezing her really hard at three- to five-minute intervals. Cut it out!
Her water breaks.	You pee all over the floor 'cause you're so stinking wasted.
The baby's head is crowning.	She gives birth right in front of you, then gingerly licks off the afterbirth, and eats the placenta so as not to give away her location to predators. (Actually, while this indicates that your wife was in real labor, it is also a sign that you married an elk.)

The "Happy Face" Chart

Some hospitals hand out the following "happy face" chart to help women and their spouses understand how far along the labor has progressed and to determine whether they should go to the hospital.

EARLY LABOR Slight discomfort. Relief that labor is starting. No need to get to the hospital, but don't go out for dinner either.

ACTIVE LABOR Moderate discomfort. It's the right time to go to the hospital. It's a bad time to play poker with her.

ADVANCED LABOR Severe discomfort. She realizes that, for the sake of the child, she'll have to stay married to you for another eighteen years. You'd better be at the hospital by now, or you'll hear about it every day until freshman orientation.

DELIVERY Very painful, but don't even think about trying to kiss it and make it better. Yuck! *You'll* need to go to the hospital if you're not at the hospital by now.

Timing Contraction Intervals

Despite the seemingly scientific precision of a "happy face" chart, the only sure way to know if your wife is ready to go the hospital is to time her contractions. To do this, you must first buy a reliable watch for yourself. Rolexes are great for this, they hardly ever break down. Why not buy one? You're wife is hardly in a position to stop you, and besides, you're doing it for her. Those Iron-Man Triathlon watches are pretty neat, too, and they have the distinct advantage of being digital, so you don't need any special skills to read them.

Assuming you have an accurate timepiece, timing contraction intervals is actually quite simple. A contraction interval begins when a woman says, "It's starting!! Oh God, help me! It's starting!" and ends when she says "It's starting again!! Oh God, help me! It's starting again!" Write the time down and say, "Hmmm."

Interpreting Contraction Times

After you say "Hmmm," your wife will undoubtedly want to know what you mean. Now, if you are a professionally trained doctor, you might actually have a clue. If you're not a doctor, look thoughtfully at this book and say, "Everything seems to be progressing nicely."

You may wish to try to figure out how much time you have to get to the hospital. Use the following table to figure out how long you have until the baby is born.

CONTRACTION INTERVALS	FIRST CHILD	SECOND THROUGH FOURTH CHILD	FIFTH CHILD AND ABOVE
Every thirty minutes	You've got time, pal.	Get in the car and drive. You might make it.	Done! Enjoy your new baby.
Ten minutes	Is there anything around the house that needs spackling? If so, feel free to get right to it.	Boil the water and get some towels.	Not Applicable.
Five to six minutes	Go to the hospital. Pick up some drive-thru on the way over.	N/A	N/A
One to three minutes	Dude, you should be there by now.	N/A	N/A

Twenty

Driving to the Hospital

Once you've determined that your wife is in active labor and you need to drive her to the hospital, make the most of it. Some husbands become flustered and forget to drive as fast as possible. Don't be that man. There will be no other time in your life when your wife will allow you to drive ninety-five in a twenty-five-mile-an-hour school zone.

Fortunately, so many of the same questions about the drive to the hospital came up during my "Daddy Dearest Child-Rearing Seminars" that I was able to put together a FAQ on the subject.

FREQUENTLY ASKED QUESTIONS ABOUT DRIVING TO THE HOSPITAL

What if I get pulled over?

Who cares? You've got a woman in labor in the car. No cop in his right mind will write you a ticket. God forbid the child's head starts poking out while he's taking out his pad, and then he has to get his precious uniform all dirty with afterbirth. Hell, no! If a cop pulls you over, all that means is you get a police escort to the hospital. And that's pretty damn cool.

What if I hit a small child while racing to the emergency room?

What better time to hit a small child? Just stop and throw him in the back seat. After all, you're both going to the same place.

My car won't go very fast. What should I do?

Hey, I didn't make you buy a shit car. Don't come whining to me like a little girl just because you have no testicles. Be a man! Buy a good car, like a Chevy IROC Camaro, and impregnate your wife again as soon as possible.

I don't have a car. I have a motorcycle. What should I do?

You are so fucked. I guess you should just tell her to hop on the back and hold on. The good thing about motorcycles is that they go really fast, so you should get there quickly if you don't wipe out taking a corner at 120 miles an hour. If you have a sidecar, you should be fine, although you are extremely weird.

What do I do if my gas light is on?

Ignore it. Duh. Unless you live in Montana and the nearest hospital is 160 miles away, in which case you should fill up at a gas station on the way. Although, since you're probably pretty good at foaling pregnant mares, you don't have too much to worry about.

What do I do when I get there?
Once you get to the hospital, drop your wife off at the emergency desk. Then, make sure you MOVE YOUR CAR! Despite what you may have heard about the soaring cost of technology, parking fees are how hospitals make their money.

Twenty-one

You Made It to the Hospital. *Now What?*

After you check in, you and your wife will be moved into a delivery room. She will be in pain. You will be bored. After all, while this sort of thing doesn't happen every day (unless you're an African king with five hundred wives or a Mormon), thanks to the miracle of television you almost certainly don't have the attention span to make it through ten to twenty hours of labor without yawning.

The first thing you will notice is that your wife keeps making annoying "Owwww" sounds. Worse, she may wish to attempt a "natural" childbirth and may not want to take an epidural.

Do NOT let your wife go through childbirth without taking an epidural, unless you want to hear her yell in pain for ten to twenty hours. And if you DO want to hear her yell in pain for ten to twenty hours, you may want to think about getting some counseling, because you have some serious issues, my friend.

Passing the Time

Assuming your wife does take an epidural, the next ten hours are going to be long and relatively uneventful—right up until the doctor tells your wife to start pushing. But that's a lot of time to fill. What should you do?

According to most authorities, you should hold your wife's hand the whole time and murmur how great she's doing, pausing only to fetch ice chips for her. Of course, if you do that, you're so gay you might as well wear a skirt.

Here are a few more palatable options:

- Play a fun little word game where you say the first thing that pops into your head. Start with: "I'm not sure I can handle being a father. Your turn."
- Say you have to check the house to make sure the gas is off. Go play golf. (Important: nine holes only!!!)
- Step out to your local Oriental massage parlor for a full-release, body to body rubdown. Feel the tension drain from your body. Return in time to see the baby pop out.
- See how much medical gear you can cram into your knapsack while the staff isn't looking. You'll be surprised how much stuff you can get.
- Learn how to take your wife's blood pressure. Make sure you figure out how to release the air in the pressure cuff, or she might lose her arm.
- Wash your face in the strange, small sink that shoots water straight up into the air and looks kind of like a toilet.

- Make your wife feel at home. Watch TV the entire time, flipping channels whenever you feel the slightest bit bored.
- Play with the hospital bed controls nonstop.
- Put on a white lab coat, walk down the hall, and give some poor shmuck an enema.

Sex

Of course, one possible way to pass the time would be to have lots and lots of sex. After all, there's really no better way to relieve stress. Unfortunately, your wife will almost certainly nix the idea since she's pretty busy. So that leaves only a few options.

Banging a Nurse

Despite what you may think you know about hospitals after repeated viewings of *Nightshift Nurses,* most nurses are not attractive, lingerie-clad women with a hands-on approach toward holistic healing. In fact, many of them are burly gay men, which is fine if that's your thing. But if you're not into being on the receiving end of hours of rough man-on-man love-play, hospitals are a relatively bad place to pick up dates, as most of the women there are either having a baby or recovering from a knife fight over five-dollars' worth of crack cocaine.

Banging a Food Services Worker

Yuck! Listen up, guy: Fishnet = sexy. Hairnet, not sexy.

Banging a Doctor

Now this is doable. Female doctors are hideously frustrated sexual beings who tend to be kind of hot-looking because their type-A personalities won't allow them to get fat. Sure, a woman doctor will be repulsed by you for coming on to her while your wife is actually having a baby in the next room, but at the same time she'll be pleased because she won't have to worry so much about you wanting a long-term relationship that might interfere with her precious career.

Solo Pleasure

This guilt-free release is a great way to enjoy your hospital stay. But with all those gorgeous, sex-starved lady doctors prowling the halls, if you want to stay faithful make extra-sure you don't get caught.

Twenty-two

The Final Push

C hildbirth is a lot like taking the world's biggest growler. First there's the pleasure of making the baby (eating). Then you get fat (you loosen your belt). Then you feel labor pains (gas). Then you go to the hospital (sit on the toilet). Then you wait (read the paper). Then you push, baby, push.

If you've ever eaten so much at an all-you-can-eat Shakey's that they've politely asked you to leave, then you know how much work that final push can be. I like to squeeze grip strengtheners in both hands when I really bear down. And, not surprisingly, when I take a big dump like that, I prefer to be alone.

Women are weird, though. They like to have you in the room when they give birth (although not when they take a load off in the shitter—go figure).

Nonetheless, when you remember how much effort it takes to knock out a really big, brown ass-sausage, you'll begin to feel the empathy necessary to helping your wife through the final stage of delivery.

Coaching

At this time, more than any other, you will be called upon to be your wife's "coach." That's fine, but if you're going to be a coach, then *be* a coach.

- Wear a red Bobby Knight sweater. Insist that everyone in the delivery room call you "coach."
- Diagram how you want the delivery to proceed on a clipboard.

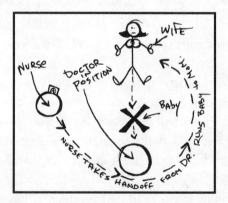

- Use an elaborate series of hand signals to indicate when and how your wife should breathe. If your wife gets confused or tired, walk up and hold a conference with her and the doctor. Tell her inane generalities such as "stay focused, but don't overthink." Despite obvious parallels to baseball, do not refer to your wife as "the mound."

- Scream at your wife constantly. Berate her for not giving 110 percent.
- Throw a chair at the doctor.

Coaching Styles

Choose the right coaching style for your personality. After all, we're not all Vince Lombardi (although the world would be a much better place if we were). Some of us are more laid-back. Others are downright lazy.

Use the following list of coaches to find a role model that's right for you.

LANDRY

Wear a hat throughout the delivery. It's that easy, and it looks so cool.

LOMBARDI

Set a time goal and stick to it. Slap her around if you have to. If your wife delivers even a few seconds late, stuff the child back in and tell her to try again—and this time, do it right.

HEINHOFLE

Who? My elementary school gym teacher, that's who. He once told me to "walk it off" after I broke my right leg. Other words of advice included: "Your family is here [hand at eye level], your schoolwork is here [hand at chin level], wrestling is up here [hand as high as he could reach]." Tell your wife to "pack up her diapers and go home" if she whines too much about the pain.

CARLESIMO
Hurl abuse at your wife in order to get her to push harder. Reminder: Keep your neck out of reach.

RILEY
Slick your hair back. Tell your wife that if anyone goes near her "painted area" she should foul, and foul hard. Later, write a book about your experience.

BERRA
Speak in charming, quirky phrases like, "It ain't over till it's over," and "I'm leaving you for a younger woman."

JACKSON
Tell the doctor to get out of the way so MJ can deliver the child. Relax.

A word on videotaping: Don't. No one wants to see your wife's yin-yang. Honest. And even if they do, they don't want to see it now, with a baby's head barreling down the pipe.

If you do decide to videotape, use a tripod. Jerky, hand-held photography may seem cool on *ER,* but really it just sucks. Think about setting up some fill lights since dark, fluorescent-green lighting only works well on the *X-Files,* and hopefully your wife isn't giving birth to anything with a tail.

To really do it right, think about using a digital camera. They cost less than five thousand dollars now, and the quality is comparable to film. With a good computer, editing is extremely easy and you can play some fun tricks like replacing your doctor's head with George Clooney's.

But far and away the best thing to do is to hire a professional actress to play the part of your wife. Unhampered by actual pain, an actress will be able to focus on giving a truly compelling performance. More importantly, as director and cameraman, you'll be able to get a close look at another woman's genitals.

If you live in southern California, I strongly suggest hiring an adult-movie star. They are much more comfortable than most "legitimate" actresses about showing their bodies on camera, and far more likely to perform fellatio for money. If you do decide to use an adult-film star, you'll almost certainly be shooting in the San Fernando Valley. Remember to drink plenty of water, as it can be extremely hot during summer.

Twenty-three

C-Sections

Y ou may be informed that, due to certain factors (the size of the baby, the position of the baby, maternal hypertension, the fact that a resident has never operated on anyone and wants to try, etc.), your wife needs a cesarean section. Don't panic! Insurance still covers it.

Indeed, C-sections are in many ways much easier than vaginal deliveries. Often they are scheduled ahead of time, which means you can take the day off from work, go golfing, and pick up the wife without any worries. And C-section babies tend to look less mangled and mushy when they come into the world. Not only that, usually the doctor will shave your wife's privates as a presurgery prep procedure. Rrrrrrrowr!

Most importantly, C-section deliveries are practically painless, so the power of your wife's guilt trips are lessened exponentially. In fact, if you get lucky, she may even feel inadequate as a mother. In that blessed scenario, you can guilt *her* into doing more and more chores as compensation for something over which she had no control. It doesn't get any better than that.

But, just because cesarean deliveries are different than vaginal deliveries doesn't mean you don't have to be on your toes. On the contrary, despite the fact a C-section is a surgical procedure, many hospitals actively encourage the husband to be in the operating room while his wife's uterus gets opened like a Ziploc bag. Don't let this happen to you! If you've ever watched one of those surgery programs on cable TV, then you know how gross an operation can be.*

THE HISTORY OF CESAREAN DELIVERIES

Contrary to popular belief, C-sections are not so named because Julius Caesar came into the world via a C-section. If that were the case, a C-section would be spelled "Caesarean." In fact, it was Cesar Romero who perfected the then-daring surgical technique in 1952 before going on to star in television's *Batman* as the devilish super-villain, the Joker.

---

* The upside of being in the operating room, though, is that you get to wear surgical scrubs and a mask. Congratulations, doctor. Yell, "Stat," as often as possible, and see how long you last before they kick you out.

Twenty-four

It's A ... live!

During the final moments of delivery, the doctor will gently help the child come out of the vagina. At this point, you must, if you ever want to have sex with your wife again, look away. Despite any locker-room braggadocio, your nob is not anywhere near as big as your baby's head.* Once you see such a monstrous object pass through, you will never feel adequate again.†

The doctor will then turn to you and announce the sex of the child (except in China, where they will reflexively drop all female children ten or twenty times onto the hard marble

---

* Yours isn't. Mine is.

† Once again: You won't. I did. But that's because I've been uniquely blessed with a prodigious unit. It's so big that I've specifically been warned not to operate it when I'm under the influence of certain medications that cause drowsiness.

floor). You should be happy that your child is healthy. Unless, of course, he or she isn't, in which case you should curse God and sue the hospital, both of which are subjects that are beyond the scope of this book.

If the doctor says, "It's a girl," grin like you're happy, always bearing in mind that she may turn out to be a stripper who can get you into her club with no cover charge. Refer to Chapter Thirteen for more helpful counseling.

If the doctor says, "It's a boy," do not whoop and holler when you see how big his balls are. All baby boys have proportionately huge testicles. Were the ratios to remain the same throughout life, your boy's nutsack would be the size of a brass diving helmet. Be thankful that this condition is only temporary. Also, do not mistake his umbilical cord for his penis. It's not that long.*

If the doctor says, "It's a . . . live," then you've got real problems, unless you think hermaphrodites are cool. And after seeing *Tranny Granny, Part IV,* I'm inclined to agree with you.

First Contact

The doctor may ask you to cut the cord, in which case you should reply, "What the hell am I paying you for, you quack?" and make him do it. The doctor may then briefly hand the

---

* Except in certain instances. When I was a child the doctor stared for hours, trying to decide which long appendage to cut. Fortunately, due to his medical training, he was able to make the correct decision.

child to you. Prepare yourself, newborn babies are gross.

To be sure, when asked about the delivery of your child you should always give the party line: "It was the most beautiful moment I have ever witnessed in my time on this earth." But know now that you will be lying. Sunsets are beautiful. Bisexual, Swedish blondes with big boobs are beautiful. Newborn children with misshapen, bruised heads, covered with bloody afterbirth, screaming their tiny lungs out are not beautiful. The key aesthetic test: Beautiful moments don't make you want to vomit. Childbirth flunks.

If you do hold the baby, do so carefully. They are very slippery. And nothing makes for more domestic tension than a botched handoff ending up in a fumble.

After you take a brief look at the baby, it then gets shown to Mommy, who will immediately bond with it, severing any remaining attachment she has to you whatsoever except possibly as a provider of food for the child.

After this sad but almost always unnoticed moment, pediatricians materialize from out of nowhere and rush the child away to wash it, put it under a bright UV light, and insert government-ordered microchips under its skin.

The Apgar Tests

During this early stage, the pediatricians will administer the Apgar test at one minute old, and again at five minutes old. The Apgar test was developed by Dr. Virginia Apgar. Dr. Apgar was steeped in the Cabbalah and soon realized that the

Why Is My Baby So Ugly?

Many fathers can't get over how disgusting their baby looks. Well, if you spent nine months in amniotic fluid and then twelve or more hours getting squished by contractions, you'd look like hell, too. So don't panic, your baby actually may not be ugly.

You may also notice one of several common conditions that could concern you. For the most part, these are normal and temporary.

AN ODDLY-SHAPED HEAD: Just because your child has a pinhead at birth doesn't mean that he's doomed to look like Zippy forever. Babies' heads are soft and get smushed around during childbirth. Eventually, they tend to pop back into a normal shape. If at all possible, resist the urge to speed up the process by molding the child's head like a Play-Doh sculpture.

VERNIX CASEOSA COATING: Commonly called "fetus cheese," this will wash off pretty quickly. Most babies have it. While indeed edible, it does not actually taste like cheese.

LANUGO: Many babies have a covering of soft, fine downy hair over their shoulders, back, neck, temples, and forehead. This is normal and usually goes away after a few weeks. If the hair is dark, coarse, and never goes away, this is perfectly normal, too. It just means your baby is Italian.

BIRTHMARKS AND SKIN LESIONS: Many light-skinned newborns have reddish blotches on the base of the neck and on the forehead called a "stork bite" and a "salmon patch" respectively. These markings will usually disappear by the time the child is four years old. The same is true for "Mongolian spots," which are bluish-gray and often appear on the back, buttocks, arms, or thighs of dark-skinned babies. However, note that a discoloration of the scalp that causes the number 666 to appear on a child's forehead (called "the sign of the beast, Naieeee!") is permanent. It is best to kill the child immediately. If you wait, his powers will only grow stronger.

BUTT UGLY JUST LIKE ITS PARENTS: If either you or your wife is butt ugly, and especially if you both are, then there is an excellent chance that your baby's condition is permanent. Sorry.

letters of her last name* could be used to determine a child's future. "A" is for appearance, "P" is for pulse, "G" is for grimace, "A" is for activity, and "R" is for respiration. Each letter is then given a number value from zero to two, resulting in a best possible score of ten.

This standardized test, for which it is virtually impossible to find a tutor or a Kaplan course, will completely determine your child's future. Many doctors will try to assuage parents' fears by stating that any score over seven is fine, and that even babies with scores below seven usually turn out to be completely normal in a matter of time. They're lying. The following list explains what the scores really mean:

APGAR SCORES AND WHAT YOUR CHILD WILL
TURN OUT TO BE

0. Dead.
1. An exceedingly boring former vice-president from Tennessee.
2. An MTV VJ.
3. A child star on a remake of *Diff'rent Strokes*.
4. A president of the United States.
5. A sales clerk at an adult video store.
6. A professional bowler.
7. Exactly like its parents.
8. A professional athlete.

* Dr. Apgar's initial attempts to invent a foolproof predictive test using a mnemonic device that relied on her first name failed terribly, as her first name is not only long but contains the letter "V."

9. A neurosurgeon/rocket scientist/author of parody books.
10. The Unabomber.

The Apgar test never lies. For example, no matter how much money you spend on expensive private tutors, a child who scored a zero on both Apgar tests will still be dead at the end of the day. Similarly, empirical studies prove that even if you send him to a fine, moral institution like Harvard, a child with a score of ten will wind up writing wordy manifestos from a shack in Montana after mail-bombing universities and airlines for twenty years.

Twenty-five

Picking a Room

After your wife gives birth, the hospital will offer you a choice between a private or semiprivate room. Semiprivate rooms cost much less than private rooms, and insurance almost never covers the price of the upgrade. You might be tempted to save the money. Don't!

Semiprivate Rooms

A semiprivate room might as well be called an "open to the public room." If your wife had just given birth in a train station, passersby would at least have the decency to pretend to look away rather than make idle chitchat with such phrases as: "Hoo-boy, eight-and-a-half pounds! That had to hurt coming out."

You will be sorely tempted to say, "How bad can it be?" Well, take a look at who your roommates might be before deciding:

- A single, depressed woman who looks morosely at her baby and then at yours and says, "Your baby is so much cuter than mine, I wish I could just switch them," before falling into a catatonic silence for the rest of the evening.
- Crazed Ethiopians who see your baby daughter and start chanting, "Clitoridectomy! Clitoridectomy!" before trying to sell you a watch and asking if you're going to eat your cinnamon-raisin brownie.
- A strange German governess and her two Dobermans standing guard over a mother and her baby born on June 6.
- Heather and her two moms.

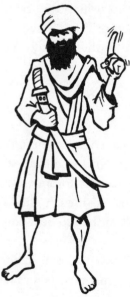

"You're shit out of luck, Mister."

- A whimpering, miserable teen and her abusive, drunken, biker boyfriend who tells you to shut up every time he hears you speak, but accuses you of plotting against him every time you whisper.

Visiting hours are extremely important in semiprivate rooms. Your roommate undoubtedly has more than ten regular visitors who crowd into your room all at once. At least four of them smell extremely bad, and one mutters to himself while idly playing with a buck knife. Theoretically, these people must leave when the visiting hours are over. In practice, these visitors speak no English. They will not vacate your room, ever. Your only hope is to yell "INS." If they're legal, you're shit out of luck.

Private Rooms

The downside of private rooms is obvious: price. Here's a helpful hint: If your wife is giving birth in Vegas, you can sometimes get the hotel to comp the room if you're a rated player. (Note: "Rated player" doesn't mean you spent an hour at the nickel slots in the hospital commissary, you cheapskate.)

If you're not a Players Club International cardholder, a private room will cost you some serious wampum. Typical rates run close to three hundred dollars a night. For that kind of cash, you could get orally serviced fifteen times by she-male prostitutes on Santa Monica Boulevard. I'm not saying that it's right for everyone, I'm just noting the difference in bang for your buck.

Private rooms sound better than they actually are. For many, the image is of an exclusive enclave of the superrich, filled with marble fountains and faithful Indian manservants. This is incorrect. For one thing, thanks to modern technology, the superrich no longer give birth to their own children. They hire surrogates to serve as their incubator units. In the near future, quantum leaps in agar technology may allow the children of the very rich to be cultivated in petri dishes.

For another, the only difference between a private room

and a semiprivate room is the absence of a deranged room-mate and her extended family. Don't knock it. It means that you won't have to Greco-Roman wrestle with a sweaty, musta-chioed Iranian for clicker control. And that's worth good money in my book.

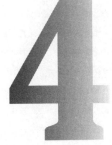

Afterbirth

Well, now you've done it. You're a father.

Some of you may think that your child is cute. Beware! That's how they sucker you in!!!! It's all a sham, a ruse. Nature programmed you to focus on the cuteness factor rather than the inescapable fact that rearing a child is a lifetime of aggravation and misery, with no reward in sight except a crashed car on prom night and a mumbled excuse about the punch having been spiked. Cute? You poor, dumb animal.

A cradle-to-college primer on how to raise your child is beyond the scope of this book, focusing as it does on the beginnings of fatherhood. Nonetheless, the following chapters should help you with the tricky first year of raising your child. As for the later years, suffice it to say that this author recommends military school as soon as possible.

Twenty-six

Keep Baby Off the Grid!!

The moment your baby is delivered, he becomes a pawn in a vast global network of multinational corporations and nation-states. Within minutes of delivery, his vital statistics will be entered in the great ZOG computer, and within thirty years he will be a wage slave controlled by the United Nations.

Why are all those interns in the delivery room? Sure, they say they're students, but in fact at least one of them is a political officer under the direct control of Kofi Annan. Think I'm lying? Ask them about it and see if they all don't nervously turn away.

Well, you're not helpless. You're the child's father, dammit, and you can stop the bastards from crushing your child's spirit before it even has a chance. And now's the time to do it. Wait any longer, and it's too late. The computer will have him cross-referenced and cross-indexed. But not yet, for now he has a clean slate. Remember, the most important gift you can give your newborn is the gift of false identity.

Fortunately, most hospitals are not used to any resistance on the part of fathers, and view the parents as foolish rubes. Thus, they won't suspect any trickery on your part. Advantage: you. The following steps will maximize your baby's chances of keeping off the grid:

1. Watch over the baby carefully, so that the UN intern will not have a chance to perform the tracker chip implantation procedure. The doctor will probably just write you a note reminding you to get your child "vaccinated," a requirement for first grade. You don't have to tell him that you plan on home schooling.

2. Give the child a common name but misspell it on the birth certificate. That way he can go through life spelling it correctly and the government will be unable to track him. Or just give him any name off the top of your head. See if the government will ever be able to find your boy when the name on his birth certificate reads "Sarah Conner."

3. Avoid giving any kind of physical evidence. Do not give stem cells, which, while theoretically useful in fighting cancer, are undoubtedly more useful as genetic markers for a universal DNA database, which will be used to identify potential organ donors for ailing world leaders.

Twenty-seven

The Great Circumcision Debate

Y es, you should get your boy circumcised since it makes for a cleaner penis,* and since, for most men, anything that even slightly diminishes sexual pleasure is a welcome change from ejaculating as soon as they're anywhere close to a vagina.† Also, it does not scar the baby mentally and people who say otherwise are big pussies who should shut up.

Debate over.

---

* Fact: people from France ("French people") tend not to have their penises circumcised, and they are notorious for their smelly, smegma-encrusted penises.

† Fact: the average time from penetration to ejaculation in America is under two minutes. I, a circumcised man, however, last until the woman is completely spent from her long string of multiple orgasms, at which point I finally allow myself and her complete release.

Twenty-eight

Other Body Modification Rituals

Apart from male circumcision, which all reputable experts agree should be done, there are a number of other cultural rituals that are best performed while the child is still a baby. While this author views any culture other than American as savage and backward, he has included a brief survey of some of these practices, figuring that some of you New Age types who called your kid "Raincloud" might be interested.

Maravi Lip Plates According to Dr. Livingstone, African Maravi tribeswomen "are in the habit of piercing the upper lip and gradually enlarging the orifice until they can insert a shell. The lip then appears drawn out

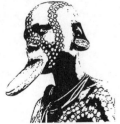

Say, "Rubber baby buggy bumpers" three times fast.

beyond the perpendicular of the nose, and gives them a most ungainly aspect. . . . These women want to make their mouths like those of ducks."
Recommendation: No.

Brass Neck Rings Married Ndebele tribeswomen use tightly fitted, constrictive, brass neck rings to elongate their necks and achieve a graceful line highly prized among their people. To the Western eye, however, they look like "bobbing head" figurines run amok.
Recommendation: No.

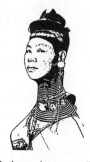

Ndebele necks can walk down stairs alone or in pairs.

Maori Facial Tattoos The Maori of New Zealand are noted for their intricate, geometric facial tattoos that empower them with perceived boosts to their courage and ferocity. Such prominent ink-work typically imposes a "glass ceiling" in the corporate world, however.
Recommendation: No.

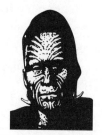

Human Resources' worst nightmare.

Full-Body Tattoos Japanese gangsters (or "Yakuza") adorn their bodies with elaborate tattoos. Often the intricate designs

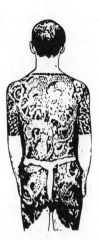

Japanese skin art on display at the Oil of
Olay museum in Amsterdam.

of dragons and the like cover the entire body except for the
hands, feet, and face. Too often, however, the practitioners'
skin is displayed in sordid, glossy tattoo magazines and, post
mortem, in strange wings of natural history museums.
Recommendation: No.

Prince Albert The body piercing of
choice among disgruntled American
gothic boys, a "Prince Albert" hoop
through the penis serves as both a
wonderful icebreaker with girls, and
a great way of flouting authority and
"sticking it to the man." Nonetheless, the resultant spray of urine
makes toilet training next to impossible.
Recommendation: No.

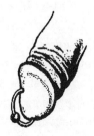

I bet Prince Albert wishes he
had stayed trapped
in that can.

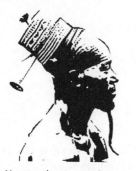

You can leave your hat on.

Head Shaping In the early 1900s, the Mangbetu people of northeastern Congo bound their babies' heads with thread in order to shape them into distinctive cones. Head shaping was also widely practiced throughout the Americas. Plateau Indians in Idaho flattened their babies' foreheads by tying the baby tightly to a cradleboard. The most famous of these tribes was called the "Flatheads." While this may have been aesthetically pleasing, unfortunately it conferred no immunity to smallpox-ridden blankets. No one alive today finds a pointy head beautiful.

Recommendation: No.

Chinese Foot Binding Despite the obvious advantages of having a child with severely limited mobility, foot binding also attracts a lot of foot fetishists who are into extensive toe shrimping and foot worship. Those people are just plain spooky.

Recommendation: No.

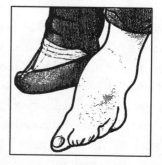

Somewhere, someone is masturbating to this photo right now. Unsettling, isn't it?

All of the Above A child with Maravi lip plates, Ndebele steel neck rings, Maori facial tattoos, Japanese full-body tattoos, the bound feet of a China doll, a Prince Albert piercing, and the pointed head of a Mangbetu tribesman would truly make an unforgettable impression, and could probably end up on Fox TV.

Recommendation: Yes.

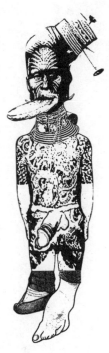

That's my boy!

Twenty-nine

The First Days Home

When you leave the hospital and arrive home, you may be tempted to treat your wife well, preparing her breakfast and running errands for her. After all, she's just been through a very tiring and painful experience, and she looks like hell.

Don't!

The first few days at home after delivery set the tone for the rest of your life as a father. If you decide to "be nice" now, that decision will haunt you for the rest of your married life. Sure, she could use a hand with the housework. But if you make the bed, then don't be surprised if five years from now, you are still making the bed. At which point, you might as well wear a French maid's outfit around the house because you, sir, are a sissy-boy.

No. Lay down the law and lay it down hard now, while she's weak. Did the shower get all mildewy while you were in the hospital? I bet it did. Give her a scrubber, some yellow rubber gloves, and some Tilex. You've got some networking to catch up on. Off to the golf course.

What about the baby? Precisely. Men aren't meant to be nurturers by nature, they're meant to hunt and gather. Unfortunately, in today's urban society, hunting and gathering is harder to accomplish than in years past (although if you go to the zoo after hours you can probably bag an elephant pretty easy). Nonetheless, you shouldn't be left alone with the child lest your ancient biological imperative drive you out of the house and into the nearest Hooters.

Holding the Baby

Should you ever hold your child? Despite the initial frisson of horror felt by all men who have ever dropped a football (the most precious of all objects), the answer is a resounding "yes!" Why?

Well, if you thought holding a cute, little puppy in your arms was a chick magnet, wait till you get your hands on a baby! Women are irresistibly attracted to a man who knows how to hold a baby without damaging it. If you're really looking to score, try strolling down a city street with a cherubic infant in a BabyBjörn Chest Papoose, while walking a golden retriever puppy at the same time. Women will hurl themselves at you like batteries at an outfielder in Shea Stadium. Bring protection!

Best of all, holding an infant is incredibly easy. Just support the child's head so it doesn't snap off like a twig. Make cooing noises if you want extra credit.

Be extremely careful, however, when patting the child gently on the back. While it looks extremely caring and thoughtful, and thus sexy, you must not forget that little babies are vomit machines. Sure, it's called "spit up," but that glob of white gunk running all over your shirt is puke, plain and simple.

Of course, babies spit up even when they are not being patted, so it's important to limit the time you are actually touching your child. Remember: A baby is like a ticking bomb. Each moment you hold your child is another moment it might explode. Pass it back to Mom as soon as you feel that enough time has passed that she won't think you're playing "hot potato" with her little darling.

Feedings

One simple rule. Mama feeds baby.

Do NOT let Mom try and foist a bottle onto you and make you feed the child during the night. Practice shouting "No" at a mirror if you think there's even the slightest chance you might cave in to her hideously unreasonable demands.

If you do collapse and agree to feed the child during the night, botch it up. One night of not eating won't hurt the child too much, and it will grant you hours of blessed sleep in the future. If your wife has any maternal instinct at all, she'll rush in to feed the child after hearing him cry incessantly while in your care. Job well done, Dad.

If she doesn't rush in, of course, there's no hope for your children. Leave her and start a new family. Write this one off as a total loss. Remember to enjoy lots of casual sex with young actresses who think that you're a producer before you settle down again. If you don't, you'll regret it.

The Breast Pump

Breast feeding offers one advantage. It makes Mom the baby's food supply and keeps you off the hook during middle-of-the-night feedings. Unless your wife figures out that she can make bottles of milk in advance using a breast pump. Do not let her do this! Sabotage the pump at all costs.

One other word of caution, while the concept of a machine whose sole purpose is to gently suck for hours on end may sound appealing to you for your own personal pleasure, beware. The pump will give you an incredibly painful hicky. Or so a friend told me. I personally wouldn't know about the agonizing pain of a "willy raspberry."

Diapers

With the advent of easy-to-use sticky tabs, changing diapers is not very hard. But it is still plenty unpleasant. The diapers, after all, contain poopy. And babies usually pee only at the exact moment that a diaper comes off. Don't let this happen to you. The appropriate way to change baby's diaper is to:

1. Release the sticky tabs.
2. Take off the diaper.
3. Drop the diaper face down on the carpet.

4. Curse loudly.

5. Leave the room and let Mom finish up.

She will never want you to change diapers again. Remember, passive-aggressive child rearing is a fantastically powerful tool. Use it to your advantage.

Pretending That You Read Those Baby Books Your Wife Gave You

By the end of the first day home, your wife will ask at least one seemingly innocuous question about the baby's general health. Beware!!! It's a trap!

She remembers all too well how, in a moment of weakness during the third month, you promised to read *What to Expect When You're Expecting*. Now she's testing you, hoping to prove what she knows in her heart to be true: that you are a fraud and a charlatan, worthy only of derision and debasement for the rest of your life.

Don't prove her correct by admitting that you never read the stupid book! And don't even think about trying to actually settle down and flip through it. Your wife has as much chance of memorizing the *New Bill James Historical Baseball Abstract* as you do of making it through more than one page of *What to Expect*.

Your only hope is to lie, bald-faced and unashamed. Simply tell her you did read *What to Expect* and here's what you learned:

- Our baby is a genius, far ahead of his peers.
- The baby's first bowel movements are a weird color because he's passing meconium out of his system. Remember: It's meconium, not zirconium. Zirconium is what she's wearing on her finger. Never say the "Z" word out loud around women.
- Though it seemed impossible, the line drawings of pregnant women on every chapter opener were less erotic than the fat hippie guy from *The Joy of Sex*.

If your wife ever catches you saying something that the authors of *What to Expect* disagree with, all you have to do is repeat this magic phrase: "Oh yeah? Well that book said that a baby's first smiles are caused only by gas. But just look at our little angel! So help me, she's smiling because she loves her mommy!" Hand the child to your wife while cooing loudly. Then flee.

Time Alone with the Child

Sometimes, despite your best efforts, you will be called upon to spend time alone with your child. Don't just sit there sullenly. That's bad for the child's psyche. Use this time constructively. Help teach the child to talk by repeating: "Dada good, Mama bad."

Thirty

Postpartum Depression:
Hers and Yours

S upposedly, many women experience terrible depression after they give birth. But who can tell? Women are moody, mysterious creatures who are best avoided unless they're drunk and horny.

As for men, all dads feel extraordinarily depressed after their child is born. Confronted with a living, breathing child, many men finally realize that the pregnancy has not just been some terrible nine-month-long, sexless nightmare that they can wake up from at the break of day. Other more thoughtful fathers will barely notice the birth, having already fallen into a numb state of mute horror when their wife announced she was pregnant in the first place. Even the truly moronic, those who thought of a baby as a wonderful gift of unadulterated joy, will find their dreamworld crashing down around them as their newborn screams and screams at three o'clock in the morning.

Fortunately, there are a number of time-tested coping strategies that will soon make most fathers much happier.

Coping Strategies

Beer

Nothing takes the edge off of fathering like an ice-cold frosty one. Sure, the little one is crying and your wife's riding your ass for leaving the boy in the crib all day, but how nice is that golden brewski? To really enjoy it, why not head down to the local public house and wash your problems away with some friends. Pretty soon, you might become as happy as that lovably raffish Andy Capp.

Check Out NBA Salaries

No matter what the players' union says about salary caps, those guys get paid a buttload. There's no reason why your kid can't become an NBA superstar. Worried that your little man won't jump high? Look at Larry Bird. That he'll be too small? Look at John Stockton. That he might be an irresponsible punk who fathers kids out of wedlock in every city he ever sets foot in? Not a problem. Just make sure you drop off the child at the park every morning and pick him up as night falls. You should be collecting some "mad bank" in about twenty-one years.

Play Golf

Don't want to count on your kid making it big and then floating you through the rest of your life? Sensible man. Take matters into your own hands. There's big money waiting to be gobbled up on the senior tour. If you're thirty now, that means you've got twenty years to get good at hitting a small, stationary ball into a larger hole with a stick. How hard can that be?

And the best part is that playing golf eats up at least six hours of your day when you include drinks at the nineteenth hole.

INTERNET PORN

Log on, then "log off." Don't ever pay for it, though. There's a lot of free porn out there. Try to find all of it. Make sure you don't miss that photo of the woman fellating a horse. It may not be erotic, but it's sure to bring a smile to even the sourest puss.

ACTUALLY INTERACT WITH THE CHILD

Some fathers report that playing with their child is satisfying and fun. Some "men" also reportedly enjoy Michael Flatley's *Lord of the Dance*. Go figure.

MARRY A TROPHY WIFE

Out with the old and in with the new. Leave your ex-wife with the hassles of child rearing. You show up every weekend to play with the child, then go home to bang your new wife—a sizzling-hot, ex-cocktail waitress. The only downside: Alimony payments can bring on symptoms very similar to postpartum depression. Worse yet, eventually your second wife will turn into an even more aggravating version of your first and the cycle will start all over again.

TELEVISION

Every day, I thank God for the blessing of twenty-four hours of cable programming available each day of the year. You should, too.

Thirty - one

Birth Announcements

A fter your child is born, you are meant to send out announcements to your friends and family relaying the
happy news. Of course, some lucky people (parents of
octuplets, parents of a boy with the head of a bat, a Kennedy,
etc.,) are excused from this tiresome chore. But assuming
your child's delivery has not been reported in *The Weekly
World News,* you have an obligation to send out an embossed
card with a pink or blue ribbon that states Baby's full name,
time of birth, place of birth, and weight.

Typically, a birth announcement looks like this:

John and Jane Public
are pleased to announce the birth of their son,
John Quincy,
on April 1, 1999
at the UCLA medical center.
8 pounds, 8 ounces

Slightly more informal, but also acceptable is this:

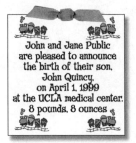

Unacceptably informal:

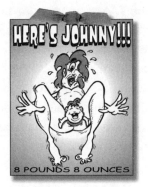

The History of the Birth Announcement

The baby shower is over. You have a phone. Why bother sending out the announcements?

Traditionally, childbirth was much more risky than it is today. Most women in the 1800s died of giving birth (as opposed to today, where the leading cause of death is elderly women having affairs with swarthy pool-boys who are much too young for them). Birth announcements, therefore, served a dual function—they announced the child's birth, and invited the recipient to console the bereaved husband.

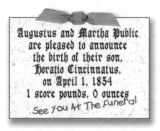

Augustus and Martha Public
are pleased to announce
the birth of their son,
Horatio Cincinnatus,
on April 1, 1854
1 score pounds, 0 ounces
See you At The Funeral

They were also particularly useful since people didn't have phones or cars, so getting the word out was a big pain in the ass. If you wanted to tell the in-laws, then you'd probably have to ride for two days and then spend the week at their place. Better to just send a note.

Even today, the birth announcement retains some usefulness. Rather than talking to your wife's father, who has a drinking habit and resents you for having deflowered his precious daughter (despite the overwhelming amount of evidence that she slept her way through the high school football team before you even met her), you can send a note and avoid those awkward minutes of sullen silence on the phone.

Also, if anybody forgot to cough up a gift for the baby shower, the birth announcement often serves as a reminder to move their sorry ass over to Baby Gap. Some older folks forget and get guilt-tripped into giving twice. That's okay, too. The rule of life has always been that the strong and young prey upon the weak and infirm.

Bringing Birth Announcements into the Modern Era

Birth announcements are not mired in the past, and new conventions are arising for conveying important information in the announcement that past generations may not have had to deal with.

For instance, the ribbon. In the past, pink meant "girl" and blue meant "boy." Ever since the advent of the red AIDS ribbon, however, ribbons can mean many things. For instance, a pink ribbon may still mean that you're having a girl, or it could mean that the parents are gay:

Gloria and Betty Public
are pleased to announce the birth of their son,
John Quincy,
on April 1, 1999
at the West Hollywood medical center
8 pounds, 8 ounces

And a yellow ribbon may mean that your child was born in captivity.

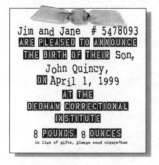

Jim and Jane # 5478093
ARE PLEASED TO ANNOUNCE
THE BIRTH OF THEIR Son,
John Quincy,
ON April 1, 1999
AT THE
DEDHAM CORRECTIONAL
INSTITUTE
8 POUNDS, 8 OUNCES
in lieu of gifts, please send cigarettes

It's not just ribbons. In today's world, family lawyers may insist that certain legal language be included in the announcement.

From the law offices of
Brykman, Duncan and Murray
10850 Wilshire Blvd. Suite 1601
Los Angeles Ca, 90218
John and Jane Public
are pleased to announce
the birth of "their" son,
John Quincy,
on April 1, 1999
at the UCLA medical center.
8 pounds, 8 ounces
PATERNITY TEST PENDING

Make Her Do It

The most important thing to remember about birth announcements is to make your wife deal with them. Picking out the right card, writing the hideously boring copy, then addressing and sending out all the cards is a ton of work. Woman's work.

Ensure that she agrees by writing your own sample announcement:

STICKEM NOTES

OOOPS! We hAD A BABy!!!
JIM + JANE PubLic
ARE PLeASeD to ANNOUNCe
the BiRth of theiR soN
JoHN QuiNCy
oN APRiL, 1, 1999
JANe hAD GoTTeN So PoRKy
Recently thAT we CouLD
baRely tell she wAs "pReggeRS"
AND She is So DAMN loose thAt the BaBy
PRACTICALLy hiT his heAD oN the FlooR,
He fell ouT So FAST
8 PoUNDS 8 ouNCeS

She'll cave in quickly. And after the child is born, she'll have nothing better to do than write out some addresses. You should offer to take them to the post office. After all, you don't want to be accused of not doing your part. And going out into the open is a man's job. Besides, there's almost certainly a strip club you can hit on the way back.

If Your Child Is the Chosen One

If you are convinced that your child is destined for extraordinary greatness, then you must write the birth announcement yourself. Your wife will just botch the job with a standard card, whereas the chosen child should probably have one that reads like this.

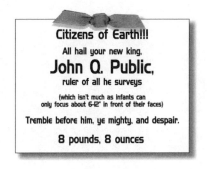

Citizens of Earth!!!

All hail your new king,

John Q. Public,

ruler of all he surveys

(which isn't much as infants can only focus about 6-12" in front of their faces)

Tremble before him, ye mighty, and despair.

8 pounds, 8 ounces

Thirty-two

Day Care Providers

Most American families rely on some form of day care to look after their children while both parents work. The parents tend to feel terribly guilty about having to return to work. They should—they are horrible, horrible, selfish people. Of course, the people who do stay at home to look after their kids are lazy, worthless dullards with no cash.

Once you decide to dump your kid off someplace so you can get on with your life, you still have to decide what kind of day care provider to choose. There are a surprising number of options.

Traditional Group Day Care

Also known as "Darwinian" day care, traditional group day care consists of a large number of children supervised by a few bored adults who occasionally dispense food and change diapers. The children soon establish a pecking order among themselves. Usually, a leader emerges and by the end of the year the older children take part in "activity circles" chanting, "Kill the pig! Drink its blood!"

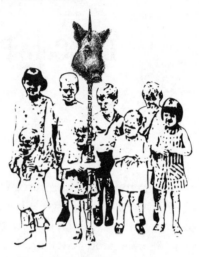

Of course, not all traditional day care centers are as good as others. Use the following checklist to help you find the best group care center in your area.

BROWN'S 10-POINT GROUP CARE CHECKLIST

1. Is the day care center licensed, as opposed to a fly-by-night "pirate" day care center?

   Y   N

2. Is the day care facility clean, with relatively little feces smeared on the walls?

   Y   N

3. Are there fresh bloodstains anywhere?

   Y   N

4. Do any of the staff members have criminal convictions?

   Y   N

5. Acquittals?

   Y   N

6. Are any of the staff members extremely hot, bisexual Swedish women?

   Y   N

7. Do the children look glassy-eyed, drunk, or sedated?

   Y   N

8. Is there at least a three to one infant to teacher ratio?

   Y   N

9. Is there a three to one spooky old guys in hooded robes to infant ratio?

   Y   N

10. Does it cost a lot?

   Y   N

INTERPRETING YOUR RESULTS:

If the answer to question 10 is yes, then you must find a cheaper place. The rest of the questions are irrelevant. Except for question 6. You can't put a price on eye candy.

Group day care centers tend to have child-rearing philosophies. Despite the fact that the best thing for infants is to roll a ball around, play with keys, or just drool while making nonsense syllables, many day care directors have master's degrees. Rather than admit that spending two years of their life learning to play patty-cake was time misspent, directors often develop philosophies of early education and couch their ideas in arcane language. Fortunately, once you understand the terminology involved, the concepts prove graspable even for a three-year-old. The most common terms are defined in the following "Day Dare Dictionary."

A DAY CARE DICTIONARY

"Emergent Curriculum": Whatever "emerges" into the teacher's head at that moment is the curriculum.

RIE: RIE emphasizes not putting too much stimulus on infants. Teachers should not do anything. Staring at the ceiling is more than enough. Soothing New Age music may have the children believing that Yanni is their father. That's okay, he seems like a nice man. While no one can actually remember what RIE originally stood for, currently the acronym means "Rest the Infant and Escape (to the teacher's lounge)."

Redirective Discipline: We redirect our ass away from the screaming kids and wait for them to work something out. If they yell too much, we eventually snap and "redirect" them with the back of our hands.

A "Nurturing Environment": You should withdraw your child immediately. They might as well have a sign that reads "NAMBLA Approved."

NAMBLA: The North American Man-Boy Love Association.

Disease Alert!! Be aware that group day care centers serve as a breeding ground for germs. If one child gets a cold, then within two days your child will have a cold. If one child gets flesh-eating bacteria, then don't be surprised when your child comes home with his skin flaking off his body. If one child gets leprosy, then, well actually you should be okay, since it takes an awful long time for leprosy to pass from person to person.* Hopefully, the school will quarantine the other kid before he can spread his disease through the dread touch of his nerveless, rotting flesh.

For this reason, it is vital that your child not go to a day care center filled with the sons and daughters of healthcare professionals. Those people catch all kinds of weird, drug-resistant diseases in the hospital, which they pass along to their kids, who in turn infect your kid, who in turn infects you. Better to send your child to a really poor group care center, where the only problems are substance abuse and violence.

Nannies and Au Pairs

The idea of having an extra woman (quite often a young, Swedish student) around the house sounds appealing. Don't fall into this trap! Nannies tend to be sexless, old Hispanic women, who teach the child to speak "Spanglish" and listen to Ricky Martin albums. Ay yai yai! If you ever fire them, they'll pretend to fall down and sue you for everything you've got. If you don't fire them, you'll end up audited by the IRS and fined for not paying the Nanny Tax. You can't win.

If you hire a sixteen-year-old English nanny, you'd better

---

* Warning for Texas residents! Besides humans, armadillos are the only other animals known to contract and pass on leprosy. Make sure that your child's day care facility does not keep a caged, leprous armadillo for the children to play with.

make sure your child does his neck-strengthening exercises every day if he's to have any hope of surviving the bouts of vigorous head shaking that will be inflicted upon him whenever he cries. This barbaric folk remedy, known throughout the world as the "British Lullaby," may explain some, if not all, of the behavior of the Royal Family.

As for the hot, young Swedes—since they're all bisexual, most of them stay in Sweden (where they are surrounded by an entire nation of tall, blond bisexuals). Only the ugly ones leave for the United States. Of course, if you happen to be the ambassador to Sweden, by all means get a nanny, but this is rather specialized advice that applies to very few of us.

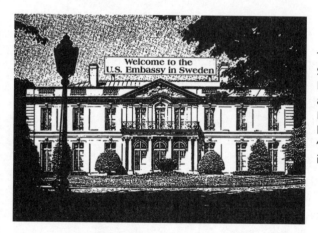

The U.S. embassy in Sweden, quite possibly the biggest plum assignment in the Foreign Service and headquarters of the "Hot Tubs for Peace" initiative.

Home Care

Home care just means you are leaving the child with a neighbor who's got a bunch of brats herself and wants to make a few extra bucks. The price tends to be much cheaper than traditional group care but remember, the woman in charge is completely unqualified and just sits around the house moping about what a shit her ex was and watching *Jerry Springer* all day. Of course, this is probably exactly what your wife would do if she stayed at home watching your child, so in that sense it's a very responsible option.

Home care facilities often have problems that traditional group settings don't have. Be aware of the following special conditions:

- Is there a dog?
- Has it been bred for fighting?
- If so, is it at least tied down?
- Is there an inbred, banjo-playing albino on the front porch?
- Do they give the children strict instructions to never, ever go into the attic?
- Is there a crystal meth or "crank" lab in the house?
- If so, do the parents get a piece of the action?

Corporate Day Care

Many large corporations offer day care to the families of their employees. While this offers the advantages of parental proximity and closer supervision of the facility, do not get sucked into this trap. Corporations are in business for one thing only, to make money.

At worst, this means that during nap time, your child will be giving bone-marrow transplants to an unidentified contact in Hong Kong. The excruciating agony of such an operation renders sleep impossible, so don't be surprised if your child is super-cranky when you pick him up.

More likely, though, the corporation will pipe in subliminal messages through the PA system during sleep hours. Typically, such centers produce children who are extremely docile, to the point of being almost mindlessly compliant. While this in itself is an excellent thing, some of the other subliminal suggestions produce darker side effects. Anecdotal evidence indicates that children placed in the Home Depot day care centers often binge-purchase yard after yard of vinyl siding before they get out of elementary school.

St. Alban's School for Boys in Washington, D.C.

A very few, gifted children will actually be kidnapped by the government and sent to an ultrasecret, "black-ops" school. There, they will spin around on three-ring gyroscopes while listening to Mozart and viewing 360-degree banks of television monitors broadcasting college-level course work. These so-called "pretenders" will have the ability to assume any identity they want due to their encyclopedic knowledge. Amazingly, many of them will grow up to seem like merely arrogant, rich brats of middling intelligence who think they are good athletes because they made a lacrosse team at a Division III school. The cover is deep, very deep.

Thirty-three

Television and the Younger Child

Many parents are concerned about the influence that television may exert on their impressionable young children. These parents, to quote Kyle Bratlowski, "suck ass."

Television is a powerful learning tool, especially if you leave it on the History Channel. There, countless black-and-white documentaries about Hitler will surely inculcate your child with the moral certainty that if you invade Russia, you will end up a horribly burned corpse in a bunker. That's important stuff. Shows on the War in the Pacific will teach your child to be wary of the inscrutable enemies from the East, a valuable lesson that will be driven home with color footage of the Tet offensive years later.

Of course, some parents worry about their children getting exposed to too much violence. Fine. If you're a pacifist, there's an easy solution. Pornography. I can't remember the last time I saw anyone injured in a porno. Usually, some lady doesn't have enough cash to tip the pizza boy and one thing leads to another. Sometimes, a woman gets hooked up to a psychic dream-reading device that looks like a colander with a lot of tinfoil all over it, allowing her analyst to conclude that she's "super horny." But there is never any violence. Not like that disgusting program, *Quincy*. Somebody always dies on that one.

Video Games

Instead of letting your child sit passively in front of the TV all day, you may want to consider other, more involving, alternatives. Some psychologists recommend against television entirely and encourage children to play engrossing, interactive, first-person "shooter" video games like Doom and Quake. Most forensics experts agree, noting that children raised on such video games gain methodical target acquisition skills combined with a healthy appreciation for the value of "kill shots."

Story Time

Virtually all experts feel that spending time reading to your child is far superior to any television show. Apparently, these "experts" aren't football fans. I'd much rather watch an NFL game than read to my child. It's not even a contest.

Thirty-four

Out with the Old, In with the New: *The Second Baby*

Some very few of you (most likely the Catholics) may be reading this book in preparation for a second child. You may be worried about helping your only child make the transition to older child.

There is no need to fear. Just by using the parenting skills you've already learned in this book—denial, withdrawal, and outright hostility—you can adequately prepare your firstborn for the true horror of what is to come.

Moreover, by paying special attention to your child's fragile psyche during this sensitive time, you can reap significant emotional rewards.

Empathize with Your Firstborn

Explain to your child that you know exactly how he feels, since you yourself used to be the only child in the family. Tell him what happened to you when he was born. Explain that

"Mommy suddenly turned all her attentions to the baby, expected me to do more chores and lost all interest in sexual activities, preferring instead to make gurgling noises over a ridiculous infant—you!" Then tell the child, "See? It all works out for the best."

Unfortunately, some children will refuse to be mollified by such a cursory discussion and will break into tears.

Make the Transition Period Work for You

Don't let the sound of nervous, jealous crying upset you. With just a little effort, you can turn your older child's fear into a powerful educational tool.

Start with simple phrases like: "We'll still love you as much as the new baby, assuming you're quieter than the new baby." Then quickly move up to: "We're only going to sell one of you to Gypsies, depending on whose room is neater." You'd be surprised at how well-behaved a properly motivated two-year-old can be.

Motivate the Younger Child

Don't forget to keep the younger child from getting spoiled. Constantly mention that, barring exceptional good deeds that demand recompense, you wholeheartedly believe in the English system of primogeniture. Comment repeatedly on the many things that the oldest child can do, and worry out loud whether the younger one is "slow." Every now and then, casually let it slip that you conceived your second child solely to provide a reserve of matching bone marrow for the older sibling should such an occasion ever arise.

In no time, you'll turn your youngest child into a simpering, toadying sycophant, catering to your every whim. Delightful.

Sibling Rivalry

Second-time parents are often shocked when they find their first child hovering over the newborn infant while holding a sharp pair of scissors perilously close to Baby's jugular. They shouldn't be. It is only natural for an elder child to instantly loathe its new rival.

Fortunately, most toddlers lack the physical strength necessary to carry out their murderous desires. Whatever happens though, don't intervene! It is this Darwinian competition that weeds out the weak and infirm. While it may seem cruel at first, natural selection benefits all of us in the long run.

Explaining How Babies Get Made

Many baby books recommend telling the truth. Well, if you think your child is ready for the whole story of how "Mommy gets sloppy drunk after a few tequila drinks, so when Auntie Sue came into town and offered to baby-sit, the first thing I did was hustle your mother to a Mexican restaurant, then I poured margaritas down her throat like I was force-feeding a goose, then I drove to a darkened lane, jammed the fuck out of my finger while fumbling to unbuckle the baby seat from the backseat, then screwed her like a carpenter on crack, finishing up just before the cops shone their light on the car and made us drive home in shame," then go ahead and tell the truth.

I personally recommend the stork story.

Thirty-five

Developmental Milestones

One really fun thing fathers like to do is check out their baby's progress against standard developmental milestones, then panic when their baby is slightly behind in one area. Some experts recommend that parents use a simple two-pronged test to determine whether their child is a drooling idiot: 1) Does he drool and 2) is he really, really stupid?

Unfortunately, all babies drool a lot at first, and most don't seem too bright either, so it's hard to tell whether they're imbeciles without resorting to more specific developmental checklists. Use my Progress Chart to make sure your baby is developing normally.

BROWN'S CRADLE TO GRAVE PROGRESS CHART
By the end of three months, your baby
Should be able to:

- On stomach, lift head up forty-five degrees.
- Follow an object in an arc about six inches above the face past the midline.
- Roll over (on a steep incline).

Will likely be able to:

- Squeal in delight.
- Bring both hands together.
- Pee at the exact moment a diaper gets taken off.

May even be able to:

- Lodge a raisin so deeply into his nose as to require hospitalization.

By the end of six months, your baby
Should be able to:

- Keep head level with body when pulled to a sitting position.
- Say, "Ah-goo," or some similar vowel-consonant combination.
- Cry all damn night.

Will likely be able to:

- Object if you try to take a toy away.
- Stand while holding on to something.
- Ruin your sex life.

May even be able to:
- See dead people.

By the end of nine months, your baby
Should be able to:
- Look for a dropped object.
- Work to get a toy that is out of reach.
- Stand in front of the TV and completely block your view of the picture.

Will likely be able to:
- Walk while holding on to furniture.
- Play peek-a-boo.
- Break something you hold dear to you.

May even be able to:
- Catch Daddy masturbating.

By the end of twelve months, your baby
Should be able to:
- Walk while holding on to furniture.
- Understand the word "no," but not always obey it.
- Object when left alone in the crib for several hours while you watch adult videos in another room.

Will likely be able to:
- Play patty-cake.
- Stand alone well.
- Recognize that you are a bad father.

May even be able to:

- Whisper his first words, "Help me!" to a passing stranger.

By the end of two years, your baby
Should be able to:

- Walk alone.
- Climb up stairs.
- Piss you off.

Will likely be able to:

- Run.
- Kick a ball.
- Royally piss you off.

May even be able to:

- Shout, "No!" for an entire year without interruption.

By the end of five years, your baby
Should be able to:

- Count to ten.
- Name at least four colors.
- Use at least four colors of crayon to scrawl all over the walls.

Will likely be able to:

- Retain some semblance of control over bodily functions.
- Print some letters.
- Understand the concept of time.

May even be able to:

- Understand the concepts in *A Brief History of Time*.

By the end of ten years, your baby
Should be able to:

- Ride a bicycle.
- Defeat you in a video game.
- Sense the tension in your marriage.

Will likely be able to:

- Burp loudly on command.
- Come home after school and watch TV until you return.
- Cruise the Internet and entice fifty-year-old pederasts to send gifts.

May even be able to:

- Hack into the Pentagon's computer system and teach it how to play tic-tac-toe, thus narrowly averting a nuclear war.

By the end of sixteen years, your baby
Should be able to:

- Feel bad about personal appearances.
- Acquire a drug habit.
- Total your car.

Will likely be able to:

- Make you feel like a bad and worthless person even on the rare occasions that you actively try to do something nice.

- Masturbate compulsively.
- Play first-person "shooter" games all day long, wear black trench coats, and write bad poetry about killing parents and classmates.

May even be able to:
- Read (but don't count on it, if you've chosen public schooling).

By the end of twenty-two years, your baby
Should be able to:
- Pierce some part of the body that it would be illegal to expose in public.
- Handle a "beer bong."
- Forget you even exist, except as a source of unearned income.

Will likely be able to:
- Annul a failed "starter marriage."
- Live at home.
- Come out of the closet.

May even be able to:
- Explain why you paid for five years at a prestigious, private university, only to watch him waste it by becoming a waiter/actor in Hollywood.

By the end of fifty years, your baby
Should be able to:

- Tell your grandchildren how bad a parent you were.
- Accept a ridiculously small buy-out package as part of a corporate downsizing program.
- Locate a prostate gland.

Will likely be able to:

- Develop a drinking habit.
- Have multiple affairs in a pathetic attempt to feel young again.
- Put you into an old-age home and never visit.

May even be able to:

- Explain with a straight face how the "trickle-down" theory of economics really does benefit the poor.

By the end of eighty-five years, your baby
Should be able to:

- Retain a driver's license by memorizing the letters on the chart five minutes before taking the eye exam.
- Mutter angrily for no apparent reason.
- Hold up a grocery line for hours while searching for a phantom coupon.

Will likely be able to:

- Spend immense amounts of money on a good-looking "nurse" who is much, much too young.

- Fritter away any remaining savings or inheritance on deceptive lottery scams that require payment to collect the so-called winnings.
- Break a hip.

May even be able to:

- Retain some semblance of control over bodily functions.

A List of Recommended Baby Books

The following is a list of recommended baby books found on the World Wide Web. Enjoy.

You Were an Accident

Strangers Have the Best Candy

The Little Sissy Who Snitched

Some Kittens Can Fly

Katy Was So Bad Her Mom Stopped Loving Her

The Kids' Guide to Hitchhiking

Daddy Drinks Because You Cry

You Are Different and That's Bad

Getting More Chocolate on Your Face

Where Would You Like to Be Buried?

The Attention Deficit Disorder Association's Book of Wild Animals of North Amer—Hey! Let's Go Ride Our Bikes!

The Boy Who Died from Eating All His Vegetables

Start a Real-Estate Empire with the Change from Your Mom's Purse

The Pop-Up Book of Human Anatomy

What Is that Dog Doing to that Other Dog?

Why Can't Mr. Fork and Ms. Electrical Outlet Be Friends?

Mister Policeman Eats His Service Revolver

Things Rich Kids Have, But You Never Will

Controlling the Playground: Respect through Fear

Bi-Curious George

Mason Brown is a managing editor at NationalLampoon.com, whose primary responsibility is to inform incredulous callers that National Lampoon still actually exists, at least as a website. He is also the author of the bestselling business humor book *Who Cut the Cheese?*

Mason has a three-year-old son, "The Boy," and a one-year-old daughter, "The Girl." Much to his dismay, his wife, Karen, insists on calling them John and Alison. She also insists on nurturing them with love rather than rely-ing on her husband's expert child-rearing advice to "mold them on the wheel of pain." She strongly recommends readers of this book to view it as "a collec-tion of lies and lewd jokes that argues powerfully for the repeal of the First Amendment."

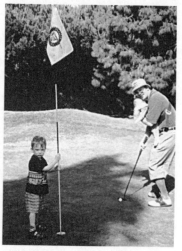

Now that Mason has both a boy and a girl, thus "completing the set," he plans to stop having babies. But he hopes to continue "trying" to have more.